the
prostate

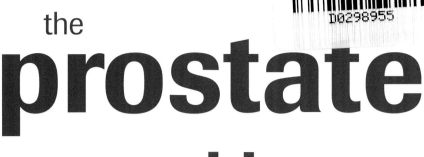

small gland **big** problem

second edition

by Roger S Kirby

Professor of Urology, St George's Hospital, London and
Chairman, Prostate Research Campaign UK

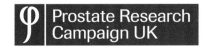

Prostate Research
Campaign UK

www.prostate-research.org.uk

The prostate: small gland, big problem
First published 2000
Second edition 2002

© 2002 Prostate Research Campaign UK

Prostate Research Campaign UK (Registered Charity No. 1037063) aims to provide information, promote education and raise funds to finance scientific and medical research into prostate disorders. Donations to further these aims may be sent to Prostate Research Campaign UK, PO Box 2371, Swindon SN1 3WJ. Tel: 01793 431901

Published by Prostate Research Campaign UK (www.prostate-research.org.uk) in association with Health Press Limited, Elizabeth House, Queen Street, Abingdon, Oxon OX14 3JR, UK. Tel: 01235 523233

Prostate Research Campaign UK and Health Press Limited have made every effort to ensure the accuracy of this book, but cannot accept responsibility for any errors or omissions.

Thanks are due to Health Press Limited for their editorial assistance and to Fine Print (Services) Ltd for their financial contribution to printing.

A note on gender
Please note that we refer to doctors throughout this book as 'he'. This in no way reflects any bias against female practitioners – this step has been taken merely to avoid clumsiness. We trust that female GPs and urologists will realize that no offence is intended and take none.

A CIP catalogue record for this title is available from the British Library.

ISBN 1-903734-27-4

Kirby, RS (Roger)
The prostate: small gland, big problem/
Roger S Kirby

Illustrated by Dee McLean, MeDee Art, London, UK.

Printed by Fine Print (Services) Ltd, Oxford, UK.

Foreword

Research has shown that doctors write about women 40 times more often than they write about men, and that they are 100 times more likely to write about children than men. It would be unfair to suggest that these figures are indicative of the place which men hold in the family or their importance to medicine. They do, however, reflect the lack of attention paid to men's ills. Nowhere is this more apparent than in the lack of interest that has hitherto been afforded to the prostate. Leonardo da Vinci in his very precise and beautifully executed 15th-century drawings of anatomy included detailed pictures of every organ, nerve and blood vessel – other than the prostate. Detailed examination of his anatomical drawings of the dissection of the male pelvis fails to show a prostate. The prostate, without which the human race would come to an end (but with which men, if they live long enough, will almost inevitably suffer problems) was ignored 500 years ago, just as it was 15 years ago.

Prostate Research Campaign UK has already done much to enlighten the general public. This book, which gives an excellent account of the prostate, should be read by medical students, doctors, and every man over 50 who, sooner or later, will almost certainly need its advice. It is another step towards enabling doctors and patients alike to be well informed so that when they discuss prostatic problems they will be speaking with knowledge, understanding, and talking the same language.

My father and both his brothers died from prostatic disease. Unfortunately there is no record of the pathology reports on my two uncles' prostates, but both died in the 1930s, in their mid-60s, immediately after surgery. My father, who was discouraged by the lack of success of his brothers' treatment, refused surgery when he developed prostatic symptoms in his late 70s. As a result, the exact nature of his diagnosis was never confirmed.

I am rather proud that, having been impressed by Roger Kirby's advocacy of PSA testing in the late 1980s, our practice became one of the first in the country to offer the test to all men over 50 who ventured through our doors as part of their annual check.

I am less proud that I only took my own advice about the need for routine PSA checks after my elder brother had developed prostate cancer. My brother always maintained that he was too busy in the City to visit doctors, but from time to time would agree to seeing his own firm's medical advisor. He had noticed that he had been becoming increasingly tired, and so visited his firm's doctor. She expressed no surprise for in her opinion tiredness was expected of a man in his late 60s who regularly worked a 16-hour day. When she found that he had a high blood pressure and an irregular heart rhythm, the diagnosis seemed obvious – he was overworked and hypertensive.

Nobody thought of taking my brother's blood for a PSA examination, and certainly no one thought of looking below the belt. About a year later my brother developed intermittent chest pain, which was induced by eating, and not unnaturally this was attributed to angina. When eventually he felt so tired and ill that he came to see me to discuss retirement, our routine PSA test gave us the true answer to his problems within an hour or two – he had a very advanced cancer of the prostate. This had spread to bones all over his body, including his breast bone – hence the chest pain after food. My brother's history is too typical. Prostate cancer is insidious in its approach – if men wait for symptoms, they wait too long.

My brother's diagnosis prompted me to follow the dictates of my own practice and immediately have a PSA test. This was indicative of a comparatively early cancer of the prostate. Within 36 hours, I had had a confirmatory biopsy. A week later, a whole-body bone scan and a MRI scan had been done and nothing untoward had been found. Within 10 days my prostate had been removed by radical prostatectomy. Although the cancer was of above average malignancy, 5 years later I remain well, still working and still enjoying my life with friends and family. I have experienced, and still experience, all the commonly reported side-effects of a radical prostatectomy, but these are a trivial price to pay for life itself.

Dr Thomas Stuttaford

Increasing prostate awareness

The foundation of Prostate Research Campaign UK dates from an idea of Tony Kilmister who contacted me in 1994 and articulated the need for an organization to fund public awareness of the increasing burden of prostatic diseases, to promote public education and to foster relevant research. Roger Kirby joined us as Chairman and Donald du Parc Braham and Jennifer Pearce as founding trustees. The organization has mushroomed since then with increasing momentum as new Trustees, such as Brian Barnes and Dr Tom Stuttaford, the well-known journalist who has contributed the Foreword, joined us together with a host of new supporters. Many of these have been recruited from the ranks of our patients but others from different parts of the country have come on board as we became more widely known around the UK. Our Annual Luncheon, the May Ball, concerts, participation in marathons and other events have grown in an exponential manner, as has our income, and are a visible reflection of our development. What makes our campaign special is the fact that we have not simply funded our own research units, but a variety of projects throughout the UK. This book, now in its second edition, is an exciting milestone in our continuing evolution. It will, I hope, also serve to bring our campaign to the attention of an increasing number of people and organizations.

Men and their partners and families often have to make difficult decisions in relation to the various treatment options available to them. Above all other objectives, I hope that this book will make this task a little easier, and complement discussions between patients and their general practitioner or urologist. There are now a number of 'self-help' books on the prostate. Some have been produced by patients and are perhaps influenced by personal experience, while others may reflect sponsorship bias. Ours, I hope, will provide a balanced, objective source of information on the three main prostate conditions of prostatitis, benign prostatic hyperplasia and prostate cancer. As the prostate rises on the healthcare agenda, increased funding is becoming available and there are many exciting prospects in the developmental pipeline, particularly in the areas of molecular biology and genetics, apart from refinements in surgical, radio-biological and pharmacological techniques. We need to build on this.

Finally, increased public awareness not only brings about earlier diagnosis, prompt treatment and better long-term outcomes, but also has the important impact of raising patient power. Healthcare budgets are not just under pressure in Britain but throughout the world. Managers, healthcare economists and politicians all too frequently reject the demands of doctors whom they may regard as having a vested interest, but are much less likely to ignore the wishes of a well-organized and informed patient lobby. Women's groups have been remarkably successful in improving health resources for women. Their menfolk need to follow their example.

Neil O'Donoghue FRCS
Consultant Urologist

About Prostate Research Campaign UK

As recently as 1994, there appeared to be a myriad of charities combating every ailment under the sun with the conspicuous exception of one – problems of the prostate. Clearly, so far as provision for prostate patients was concerned, here was a 'Cinderella' area that needed urgent attention. Prostate Research Campaign UK was born.

At the outset, we decided not to link our organization to any one particular hospital or institution so that we could enjoy the freedom to support good research anywhere in Britain. Our first research project in Edinburgh has been followed by many others across England, Scotland and Wales.

Our other principal objective, the provision of information to patients, was not neglected. A variety of fact sheets, leaflets and other literature were produced, followed by the happy cooperation with Health Press (to whom warm thanks are due) resulting in the publication of two books. This volume, the proceeds of which will go to Prostate Research Campaign UK, is intended to be even more helpful than the first edition of *The Prostate: Small Gland Big Problem*.

Up-to-the-minute information is now available on our website at www.prostate-research.org.uk and our regular newsletter, *Update*, is always an eagerly awaited publication.

All these activities cost money – a lot of money – and the ability of Prostate Research Campaign UK to pursue its goals is in direct relation to the financial support it receives. Your support will be warmly welcomed.

Anthony Kilmister
Founder, Prostate Research Campaign UK

Contents

Introduction

At the beginning of the 20th century, the average life expectancy for a man in Europe or the USA was only 49 years. As diseases of the prostate typically affect men beyond middle age, the likelihood of a man in the early 1900s suffering from one of these conditions was rather slim. Now, at the dawn of the new millennium, however, life expectancy for men extends well into the seventies, and this increased longevity has been accompanied by a rising tide of prostate disease. Over the next 20 years, life expectancy is predicted to rise still further, to 80 and beyond. What we are witnessing at the moment is, then, simply the tip of the iceberg. The number of men with either prostate cancer or benign prostatic hyperplasia is set to more than double by the year 2020.

Recently there has been a surge in public interest in the prostate, largely as the result of a spate of media attention. Scarcely a week goes by without a newspaper or television feature on this aspect of men's health. Prominent personalities, including the former Archbishop of Canterbury Lord Runcie, Sir Julian Critchley, Sir Harry Secombe and George Carman QC, have also spoken openly about their prostate problems, fuelling an already kindled fire, before sadly passing away as a result of the disease.

This increasing focus can only be good news, as men with prostate disease can be cured by a little knowledge and timely action. Men, and the women who love and support them, need to be aware of the symptoms and signs of prostate problems, and the possibilities of a simple examination and a blood test. This book contains the essence of the things that you and those closest to you need to know to respond appropriately to the threat of these widespread diseases. Use the information to obtain the best treatment for you – you owe it to yourself and those that love you.

Roger Kirby MA MD FRCS (Urol) FEBU
Professor of Urology and
Chairman, Prostate Research Campaign UK

Prostate awareness

The prostate is a chestnut-sized gland that is present only in men. It is located in the pelvis, at the exit of the bladder, and surrounds the tube known as the urethra (through which urine flows from the bladder to the outside of the body). Tiny at birth and throughout childhood, the prostate enlarges after puberty, stimulated by rising levels of the male hormone testosterone, to a volume of around 20 cc. Although small compared with other organs, the prostate looms ever larger as a potential source of disease and disability once a man passes middle age.

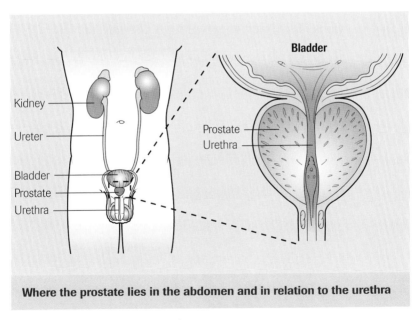

Where the prostate lies in the abdomen and in relation to the urethra

The prostate is subdivided into three zones: central, transition and peripheral (see diagram on page 4). The peripheral zone is located at the back of the prostate and is the part most susceptible to both prostate cancer and prostatitis. The third and most common prostate problem – benign prostatic hyperplasia (BPH) –

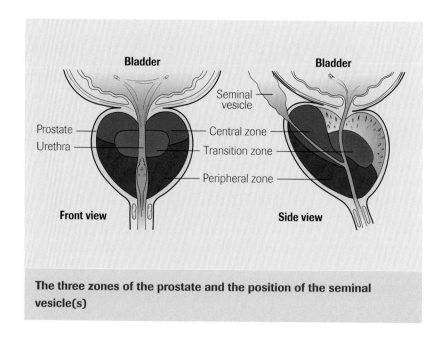

The three zones of the prostate and the position of the seminal vesicle(s)

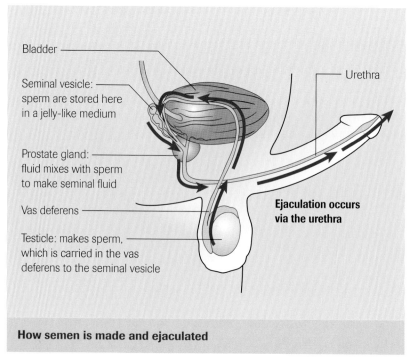

How semen is made and ejaculated

develops in the transition zone, which lies in the middle of the gland and surrounds the urethra. (The enlargement of the prostate in BPH causes pressure on the urethra, which can lead to problems with urinary flow and difficulty emptying the bladder.)

Function of the prostate

The prostate gland manufactures an important liquefying component of semen. Sperm are produced in the testicles and then stored just behind the prostate in the seminal vesicles. Here, and at the time of ejaculation, the sperm are in a jelly-like medium. At orgasm and ejaculation, the prostate and seminal vesicles contract, mixing their respective contents. The fluid in the prostate contains large amounts of a substance known as prostate-specific antigen (PSA), which liquefies the previously gelatinous sperm mixture, allowing the sperm to move freely in search of an ovum to fertilize.

Common diseases involving the prostate

Because the prostate surrounds the urethra, any disease of the gland is likely to cause disturbances in urinary flow, and in the frequency and efficiency with which the bladder is emptied. There are three common diseases that involve the prostate:

- prostate cancer, which is the second most common form of potentially lethal cancer to affect men and is likely to become the most common by 2005
- BPH, a disorder that results in frequent urination and a reduced urinary stream, and affects almost one man in two beyond middle age
- prostatitis, an inflammatory disease affecting mainly younger and middle-aged men, which is characterized by symptoms of pain and discomfort around the anus, scrotum and the area in between (the perineum).

Each condition is described in detail in later sections, starting with prostate cancer, which is potentially by far the most serious, and then BPH, easily the most common, and concluding with prostatitis which, though less serious than prostate cancer and less common than BPH, can cause distressing and debilitating symptoms among its many sufferers.

Men's health issues

All three prostate diseases – prostate cancer, BPH and prostatitis – tend to cause a greater impact on a sufferer's quality of life than is, in fact, necessary. That the conditions often reach a relatively advanced stage before men seek medical help is often the result of men's *laissez-faire* attitude to lower urinary tract symptoms, embarrassment about discussing this area of their anatomy with their doctor, and their general reluctance to undergo regular health checks.

In fact, most prostate diseases eloquently illustrate the 'stitch in time' principle. A 'window of curability' exists for prostate cancer, but once this is closed, neither surgery nor radiotherapy is likely, ultimately, to be successful. With BPH, several studies have confirmed that there is a level of secondary damage to the bladder caused by obstruction at which complete recovery becomes less likely. And if prostatitis becomes chronic, then repeated and prolonged courses of treatment are often needed.

Men's attitude towards their health has traditionally been 'if it ain't broke, don't fix it'. These days, the thinking should be more along the lines of 'if you look after your body (and particularly your prostate), it has less of a tendency to go wrong'. Regarding prostate health, regular prostate checks allow disease to be detected at a stage when it can generally be resolved, while preventive strategies may reduce the risks of disease developing in the first place. It makes good sense to combine these with regular, more general health checks to exclude conditions such as high blood pressure and diabetes, and to encourage a healthier lifestyle, particularly with respect to exercise and diet.

So when should you see your doctor?

Problems with urinating are the most common symptoms of prostate disease. Visit your doctor if you regularly experience one of the following:

- a weak, sometimes intermittent flow of urine
- difficulty starting to urinate
- a need to urinate frequently
- a need to urinate urgently (you don't feel able to put it off)

- having to go to the toilet several times during the night (for a period of time)
- a feeling that your bladder is not completely empty after you have finished urinating
- pain or burning when passing urine
- blood in your urine.

Of course, problems may develop before any symptoms arise. For this reason, it's generally advisable for most men over 50 to have an annual health check which includes an assessment of the prostate, including a PSA test.

What is, and what causes, prostate cancer?

Prostate cancer develops as a result of a progressive series of faults occurring in the genes that control cell growth in the prostate. Normally, cells divide only when the body needs them to, and the process is under strict genetic control. When this genetic control breaks down and the cells begin dividing in an unregulated manner, a mass of excess cells forms (a tumour). A tumour can be benign or malignant, depending on its capacity to invade healthy surrounding tissue (if it can invade, it is cancerous). Because of its capacity to invade surrounding areas, cancer can spread to sites around the prostate, in which case it is said to be locally advanced. It can also spread to distant sites in a process known as metastasis, which occurs as the cancer becomes more advanced. Cancer cells can break off from the tumour in the prostate and enter the bloodstream and lymphatic system (the latter is a network of tiny vessels that drain fluid from all the organs in the body). In this way, cancer cells are transported to other parts of the body (for example, the lymph nodes or bones) and, like seeds growing in fertile soil, dangerous secondary tumours develop.

Stages of cancer

The earliest stage in uncontrolled cell growth is not actual malignancy, but *pre*-malignancy, known as prostatic intraepithelial neoplasia (PIN for short). PIN is characterized by a 'heaping up' of cells within the prostate, but there is no invasion of healthy tissue at this stage. With time, however, these dividing cells may develop the ability to invade the prostate tissue. Such early signs of invasion give the pathologist looking at a sample (biopsy) of prostate tissue under a microscope the clue that actual cancer has developed from the pre-malignant PIN changes. At this stage, the level of a substance known as PSA (see page 14) in the blood can also begin to rise – another clue that prostate cancer is developing.

As cancer develops from prostate cells, under the microscope, early, less aggressive cancers bear a close resemblance to normal tissue. As the cancer becomes more aggressive and potentially dangerous, these similarities are progressively lost. This process is known as 'de-differentiation' and was described in the 1960s by the pathologist Dr Gleason. A sample of prostate tissue is given a 'Gleason grade' according to the shape, size and structure of the cells in the sample. The grading runs from 1 to 5; the higher the number, the more aggressive the cancer. Because the cells will not appear uniform across the tissue sample, the two most prominent regions are usually assessed, and the two grades added together to give what is known as the 'Gleason score'. Doctors can use this to estimate the likely outcome for their patients. The higher the score (from 2–10), the more potentially dangerous the cancer.

Once prostate cancer cells have developed the ability to invade tissue, they initially spread locally within the gland and start to

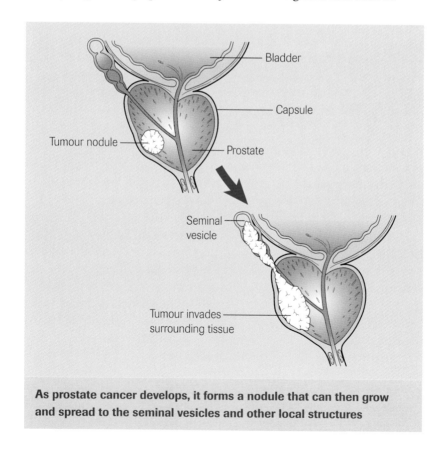

As prostate cancer develops, it forms a nodule that can then grow and spread to the seminal vesicles and other local structures

9

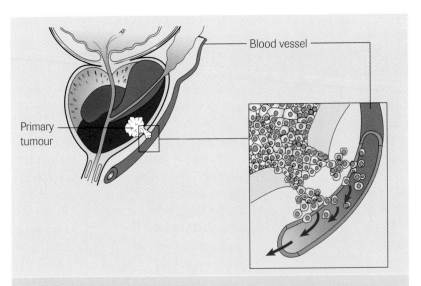

As the cancer becomes more advanced, the cells are able to break off from what is known as the primary tumour. These cells enter the blood or lymphatic system, and are transported to distant parts of the body. Once deposited at a site, the cancer cells start to grow and multiply, and new secondary cancers called metastases are formed

invade the capsule. Small tumours can be detected only by examining a biopsy of an apparently normal gland under the microscope; larger cancers can usually be felt by the doctor as a firm nodule during an examination via the back passage (rectum) known as the digital rectal examination or DRE.

At first, the cancer spreads locally to tissues around the prostate. Eventually, however, it can spread to more distant sites, such as the bones. The mechanisms by which the life-threatening ability to spread (metastasize) is acquired by the cancer cells are currently the subject of intense scrutiny. Central to the process is the ability to acquire a new blood supply to provide oxygen and nutrients to the cancer cells so that they can grow (all cells have these requirements). The development of a new blood supply has been termed 'angiogenesis', and angiogenesis inhibitors, which include the infamous drug thalidomide, as well as newer agents such as angiostatin, provide a very promising new avenue of treatment for prostate cancer.

Why metastatic prostate cancer cells show such a preference for settling and developing in bone is still unclear, but it must provide a favourable environment for them. (There is a network of veins around the prostate that drains directly into the vertebral column, which may account for the tendency of bone secondaries to occur in this site.) The cancerous nodules that develop in bone far distant from the prostate often cause pain and swelling, and sometimes fractures. Sadly, many men consult their doctor only when their cancer has reached this stage, by which time the disease can only be slowed temporarily – cure is no longer possible.

Why do some men get prostate cancer and others do not?

Overall, the lifetime risk of developing prostate cancer is around 10%. Your chance of getting prostate cancer depends on your personal risk factors. Having a risk factor makes you more likely to develop a certain disease (for example, a high cholesterol level in the blood is a well-known risk factor for heart disease).

The strongest risk factor for prostate cancer is increasing age. The disease rarely occurs in men under 40, but commonly affects men beyond this age. With the average age of death from prostate cancer in the UK standing at around 70 years, the average loss of life expectancy is about 9 years – precious retirement years for which most men have been working and anticipating all their lives.

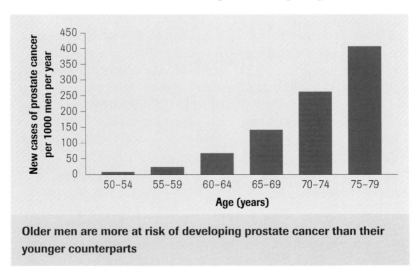

Older men are more at risk of developing prostate cancer than their younger counterparts

The next most important risk factor for prostate cancer after age is family history. Like breast cancer, prostate cancer runs in certain families and has been linked, so far, to two genes. A man whose father, brother, grandfather or uncle has had the disease has an increased risk of developing prostate cancer compared with one without an affected relative. This is particularly the case if the disease developed in the close relative when he was under 60.

Risk factors for prostate cancer

- Belonging to an older age group (usually 50+ years)

- Having a close family member who has had prostate cancer

- Having certain racial origins; for example, it is more common among men of Afro-Caribbean origin

- Following certain eating patterns, such as a high-fat diet

- Low exposure to sunlight

Race is also a factor, with men of Afro-Caribbean extraction being at highest risk. These men seem to develop a more aggressive form of the disease and at a younger age than Caucasians. Men of Far Eastern descent seem to be relatively less likely to be affected by the disease.

Clearly, you can't change your age, ancestry or race (these are 'non-modifiable risk factors'). However, several other risk factors for prostate cancer have been identified over which you can have some influence. The first of these so-called 'modifiable risk factors' is a high level of saturated animal fat in the diet. A man worried about his risk of prostate cancer (or indeed heart disease) is well advised to reduce his intake of eggs, milk, cheese, butter and red meat. In addition, various dietary supplements may offer some protection. Preliminary studies suggest that both vitamin E and selenium may help. Recently it has been reported that lycopenes which are found in tomato skins are protective against prostate cancer. The advised dose of vitamin E is 400 international units/day, selenium 200 micrograms/day and lycopenes 15 milligrams/day. (If you want to take a vitamin or mineral supplement, it's a good idea to check with your GP first; some ingredients can interfere with medicines that you might be taking, or affect an existing medical condition.)

Geographically, prostate cancer tends to become more common as you move away from the Equator; Norway and Sweden have the highest death rates from the disease worldwide. This fact points us to two further possible modifiable risk factors – low vitamin D and low exposure to sunlight, which itself helps the body to produce vitamin D.

Prevention

As already mentioned, prostate cancer is characterized by an abnormal overgrowth of prostate cells. As scientists unravel the steps involved in the development of this abnormal cell overgrowth, it is possible, and indeed probable, that we will one day be able to intervene to reverse the earliest phases of the disease. A number of compounds that have this potential are currently being investigated for effectiveness and safety. One of the problems is that it is considerably more difficult (and expensive) to demonstrate that a given drug or vitamin is capable of *preventing* a disease than it is to show that it can *cure* a specific problem once it has developed. Because we are never sure exactly who will develop a disease such as prostate cancer, very large numbers of individuals have to be studied for many years (5, 10 or even 15) before we can be certain that a drug can safely and effectively prevent the disease from occurring. At the time of writing, the drug Proscar (finasteride) is being evaluated for its preventative activity. The results of this trial are expected in 2003 or soon after. A new drug, dutasteride, which has a similar effect to that of Proscar, is also being tested in this context.

The PSA test

PSA, prostate-specific antigen, is a protein-like substance that occurs in abundance in the fluid within the prostate. Testing blood samples to determine the amount of PSA (a 'PSA test') is central to the early detection and selection of effective treatment for prostate cancer. Monitoring a man's PSA level is also extremely helpful

Prostate gland   Blood vessel

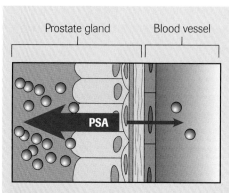

Normal

Cells in the prostate are healthy and organized in a tight pattern. Only a small amount of PSA leaks out of the prostate and gets into the bloodstream

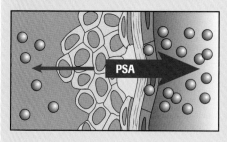

With prostate cancer

Now the cells are disorganized and the layers between the prostate and blood vessel become disrupted. More PSA can leak into the blood vessel as a result

The growth of cancer cells in the prostate disrupts the structure and organization of the tissue. PSA inside the prostate is able to leak into the nearby blood vessels more readily than it does in a healthy prostate. As a result, the amount of PSA in the blood increases, which is why measurement of PSA in a blood sample can help to diagnose prostate cancer

once therapy has been started, as it can indicate how effectively treatment is working.

Basis of the PSA test

As the pre-cancer stage PIN (see page 8) evolves into invasive prostate cancer, the membrane surrounding glands within the prostate may start to break down in small areas. As a consequence, the fluid in the prostate and the PSA it contains start to leak out. The PSA finds its way into the blood and so the amount of PSA in the blood starts to increase. Progressively worsening damage to the prostate makes it more leaky which, in turn, results in higher PSA levels. A normal PSA level (in a man with no prostate problems) is usually accepted as being below 4 ng/mL (4 nanograms per millilitre), but this rises with age so that in men over 70 a cut-off of 6.5 ng/mL is accepted (see table below).

PSA in the bloodstream is bound to one of two proteins – antichymotrypsin and alpha macroglobulin. For reasons that are still not clear, in men with prostate cancer the amount of unbound or 'free' PSA is reduced. As a consequence, a reduction of the percentage free PSA is also an early warning sign for prostate cancer. The cut-off point is usually taken as 18%; values above this indicate benign prostate enlargement, while values less than 18% increase the probability of prostate cancer being present.

When doctors and journalists talk about screening for prostate cancer, they are usually referring to the potential to test every man's PSA level at fixed intervals of time (like the smear test for women), from the age of around 50 onwards. If the test is so useful, why

Increase in accepted PSA cut-off with age	
Age	PSA cut-off
40–49 years	2.5 ng/mL
50–59 years	3.5 ng/mL
60–69 years	4.5 ng/mL
Over 70 years	6.5 ng/mL

isn't it used in this way? There are several points that have to be considered, and the pros and cons of the PSA test are summarized in the table opposite.

Issues surrounding the PSA test

Overdetection of clinically insignificant cancers
As prostate cancer occurs mainly in men beyond middle age, it is perfectly possible that a small cancer might never grow sufficiently large to cause symptoms during a man's natural lifetime. The anxiety caused by a 'positive' (high) PSA result might reduce the man's quality of life by causing unnecessary worry, whereas if he remained ignorant of his condition, his life would be unaffected. However, fears of this sort of overdiagnosis of prostate cancer have lessened as a number of scientific papers have now reported that small and insignificant cancers rarely result in a raised PSA level.

'False-positive' results
An elevated level of PSA in the blood does *not* necessarily indicate cancer. Indeed, the average PSA level rises with age and any disease of the prostate – particularly BPH, but also prostatitis – can result in an elevated PSA, though usually to a rather minor extent.

A high PSA value will usually prompt a doctor to request a biopsy, where samples of tissue are taken from the patient's prostate. However, scientific studies have shown that when samples of prostate tissue are examined under the microscope, only one man among four with a PSA value between 4 and 10 ng/mL will be found to have cancer (so three will *not* have cancer even though their PSA levels are raised).

With a higher cut-off (say PSA above 10 ng/mL), the probability that a subsequent biopsy will confirm prostate cancer rises to more than 60%. Of course, the problem with using a higher cut-off to determine who should receive a biopsy is that as the cut-off value increases, so does the 'false-negative' rate. (False negatives are men whose PSA value is below the cut-off, yet who do have prostate cancer; see the diagram on page 18. Remember that early prostate cancer can be present even when the PSA value is below 4 ng/mL.) Also, if cancer is to be identified at a stage when it is still curable, then it should be detected before the PSA rises much above 10 ng/mL.

The pros and cons of PSA testing

Pros

- Allows early detection of potentially curable prostate cancer

- May allow the doctor to estimate prostate size in a patient with BPH

- Helps the doctor predict response to certain drugs

- Allows the doctor to estimate how advanced the cancer is at diagnosis

- Can be used to monitor men at increased risk of prostate cancer, such as those with a family history

- Can help the doctor estimate the patient's risk of developing prostate cancer in the future

- A negative result is reassuring

- Helpful for monitoring response when treatment is given

Cons

- Clinically insignificant cancers may be detected, causing needless worry and further medical procedures for the patient (this appears to be unusual, however – see text)

- Men without cancer may have a false-positive result (particularly those with borderline PSA values)

- Patients may be nervous while awaiting results

- A positive result causes anxiety

- There are cost implications – not only regarding the PSA test, but of biopsy and treatment options if the biopsy is positive

- Exposes those undergoing biopsy to the risks of bleeding and infection

Anxiety before the results become available

The speed with which you get your test results depends on where you have your test. It can take anything from a couple of hours to several weeks – obviously those at the longer end of the scale have

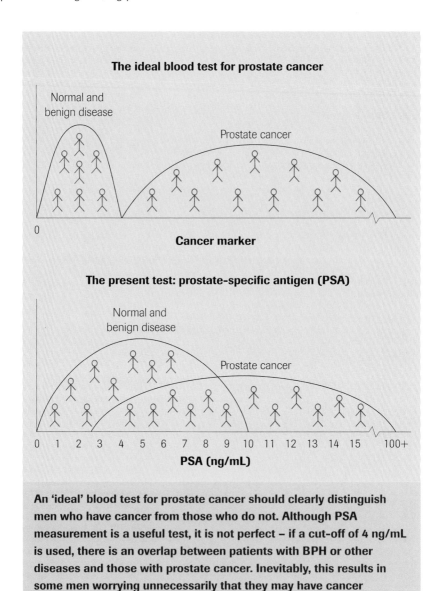

The ideal blood test for prostate cancer

Normal and benign disease

Prostate cancer

0

Cancer marker

The present test: prostate-specific antigen (PSA)

Normal and benign disease

Prostate cancer

0 1 2 3 4 5 6 7 8 9 10 11 12 13 14 15 100+

PSA (ng/mL)

An 'ideal' blood test for prostate cancer should clearly distinguish men who have cancer from those who do not. Although PSA measurement is a useful test, it is not perfect – if a cut-off of 4 ng/mL is used, there is an overlap between patients with BPH or other diseases and those with prostate cancer. Inevitably, this results in some men worrying unnecessarily that they may have cancer

more opportunity for anxiety. Ask your doctor about the usual waiting time for results in his clinic. Over-the-counter PSA tests, which will allow self-testing, are becoming available in chemist shops. Like the whole PSA issue, these home tests are bound to be rather controversial.

Exposure of those undergoing biopsy to the risk of complications

Biopsy (in which 6–12 small pieces of prostate tissue are removed so that they can be examined for signs of prostate cancer) may result in minor bleeding and the appearance of blood in the semen. This usually settles spontaneously after a week or two. There is also a small risk of infection, but doctors try to minimize this by prescribing antibiotics for you to take before and for several days after the biopsy (the procedure for a biopsy is described on pages 25 and 26). If you have had a biopsy and develop symptoms of infection, contact your doctor immediately.

It's not always cancer

It is worth re-emphasizing here, at the end of this section, that a PSA level that is higher than normal does *not* necessarily mean that you actually have cancer. Both BPH and prostatitis can result in elevated PSA levels in the blood, and your doctor will cross-check your PSA result with your symptoms, the result of a DRE and probably the results from a biopsy to make the diagnosis. If you have a raised PSA, but a negative result on biopsy, your doctor will probably monitor your PSA level over time. Depending on further results, he may suggest that you have another biopsy at a later date. The value of sequential PSA testing lies in its ability to set a baseline. A sudden or progressive rise above this level may act as an early warning of prostate cancer development.

Your choice

In the end, it's up to you whether you have the PSA test or not. But make sure you base your decision on reliable information, and not the latest newspaper, radio or TV article, or some unsubstantiated internet site. The Department of Health has recently changed its policy on PSA testing and has agreed that men should be entitled to this test once they have had enough information to make an informed choice.

A raised PSA: what happens next?

Finding a good urologist

If your GP finds that you have a raised PSA level (above 4 ng/mL), or a reduced percentage of free PSA (less than 18%) you will probably be referred to a urologist – a specialist in disorders affecting the kidney, bladder and prostate in men (and the urinary tract in women). It is vital that you feel comfortable with, and confident in, your urologist. You should understand his explanations of procedures and options, and he should be prepared to discuss fully anything that concerns you or your partner. In this day and age, don't simply accept that the 'doctor knows best' – it's your health and peace of mind at stake here, so make sure that you've had all your questions answered before you leave the consultation room. If you are not happy with your urologist, go back to your GP and discuss the matter with him. You may decide that you would like to see a different urologist. If so, tell your GP and ask him to organize this.

Alternatively, you may want to find your own specialist on a private basis. If this is the case, the first thing to do is to check your health insurance, if you have it. Some companies will not cover your expenses unless you have been referred by your GP. Also, you (or your insurers) may want to check the prices of treatment at an early stage. The clinic should provide a price list for you – if they don't, talk directly to the urologist. If you aren't happy with your service, talk to the clinic manager or the urologist (or his secretary) directly – you are a prospective customer and they will be unlikely to want to 'lose' you. If you are still not happy, go back to your GP. If you find it difficult to voice your concerns face-to-face or if you feel that you might forget some things, write a letter or list so that you can make sure that all your points are answered.

Tests

Your urologist may repeat the tests that your GP has already carried out, such as the PSA and percentage free PSA measurements. He may want to check your situation for himself; for some tests, it is important that the samples are sent to the same laboratory for analysis if you are being monitored over a period of time. The tests that you might have are outlined next.

Blood test
The basis of the PSA test was described earlier (see pages 15–19). Other results (such as your blood sugar and cholesterol level) may be used as indicators of your general health and to rule out diabetes or an abnormal lipid profile.

Urine test
You may be asked to provide a urine specimen. This could be checked for bacteria, as you may have a urinary tract infection, and/or blood. Blood can be found in the urine if the prostate cancer has spread into the urethra that runs through the prostate, so its presence is a clue to the urologist about the nature of your problem. Other important causes of blood in the urine include bladder stones and bladder cancer, so this is a finding that should not be ignored.

Physical examination and digital rectal examination
The urologist may examine you in general, but will almost certainly perform a digital rectal examination (DRE). Undeniably, it is an uncomfortable experience and one that some men dread, but is actually less uncomfortable than a visit to the dentist. Urologists perform this day in, day out, but if that does not reassure you, just keep thinking about the consequences of ignoring your condition. A few moments of minor discomfort are surely worthwhile.

Your urologist will put on a glove and apply some lubricant to his finger. He will tell you which position to adopt, probably one where you lie on your side with your legs pulled up towards your chest. He will then insert his finger into your rectum, passing through the sphincter muscle that keeps the anus closed (see diagram on next page). He will then feel your prostate, noting its size, shape, firmness and how its surface feels. The examination is not painful, just uncomfortable. Try to relax until it's over – it only lasts a few seconds.

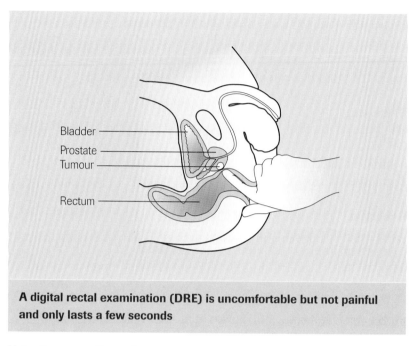

Bladder
Prostate
Tumour
Rectum

A digital rectal examination (DRE) is uncomfortable but not painful and only lasts a few seconds

Urination questionnaire

Prostate cancer may be affecting your ability to empty your bladder, or you may have BPH that is affecting your urine flow. In order to investigate your symptoms in a meaningful way, your urologist may give you a questionnaire to fill in (see opposite). You may be asked to fill it in while you are in the clinic, or you may be able to take it home with you to complete and return at your convenience.

If cancer is suspected

If cancer is suspected, your urologist will first need to check whether you do in fact have cancer. If you have, he will then need to determine how aggressive it is and how far it has progressed. You may hear a reference to the grade and stage of your cancer. These are important in selecting the best treatment for you.

Grade

This is a measure of how aggressive the cancer is. We have mentioned previously how the cancer cells in the prostate start

	Not at all	Less than 1 time in 5	Less than half the time	About half the time	More than half the time	Almost always	Patient score
1 Incomplete emptying Over the past month, how often have you had a sensation of not emptying your bladder completely after you finished urinating?	0	1	2	3	4	5	
2 Frequency Over the past month, how often have you had to urinate again less than 2 hours after you finished urinating?	0	1	2	3	4	5	
3 Intermittency Over the past month, how often have you found you stopped and started again several times when you urinated?	0	1	2	3	4	5	
4 Urgency Over the past month, how often have you found it difficult to postpone urination?	0	1	2	3	4	5	
5 Weak stream Over the past month, how often have you had a weak urinary stream?	0	1	2	3	4	5	
6 Straining Over the past month, how often have you had to push or strain to begin urination?	0	1	2	3	4	5	
7 Nocturia Over the past month, how many times did you most typically get up to urinate from the time you went to bed at night until the time you got up in the morning?	0	1	2	3	4	5+	
Total score							

	Delighted	Pleased	Mostly satisfied	Mixed	Mostly dissatisfied	Unhappy	Terrible
Quality of life due to urinary symptoms If you were to spend the rest of your life with your urinary condition the way it is now, how would you feel about that?	0	1	2	3	4	5	6

A sample questionnaire on urinary symptoms

out looking very similar to normal prostate cells, but start to de-differentiate (i.e. become more aggressive) as the cancer progresses (see page 9). Grading is a means of assessing this process in a standardized way, and is performed in a laboratory by specialized pathologists.

The most common grading system is the Gleason system. From incidental post-mortem findings, we can speculate that grade 1, 'latent', prostate cancer is probably quite common among men aged over 40; these small tumours can grow very slowly, and so many men will never develop symptoms during their natural lifespan. However, a cancer that progresses more quickly (that is, a more aggressive one) will show a less differentiated pattern, and will be graded more highly. The cancerous areas in the prostate may vary and have different grades, so the grades of the two most prominent areas are added together to give a Gleason score (for example, 3 + 4); the maximum is 10 (5 + 5). This figure then gives your doctor an idea of how quickly your cancer is likely to progress and therefore helps him advise you about treatment.

Gleason score and the risk of prostate cancer progressing

Gleason score	Risk
2–4	Low
5–7	Medium
8–10	High

Stage

The cancer can also be classified according to how far it has spread, that is its 'stage'. The tumour–nodes–metastases (TNM) system is commonly used, and involves the doctor assessing how far your cancer (tumour) has spread in and around the prostate, whether it has spread to the nearby lymph nodes (nodes) and then whether it has spread (metastasized) to the distant lymph nodes and bones. Knowing the stage of your cancer helps your urologist to decide on the most appropriate course of action.

Grading and staging tests

PSA measurement and DRE are both important for staging cancer, but you will almost certainly have to undergo some further tests.

Ultrasound

This may be used to assess the size and texture of the prostate; the specific technique is called transrectal ultrasonography (or TRUS for short). A lubricated probe is inserted into the rectum, where it passes high-frequency sound waves through the prostate. Computer analysis of the echoes, which vary according to the density of the material the waves are passing through, can produce

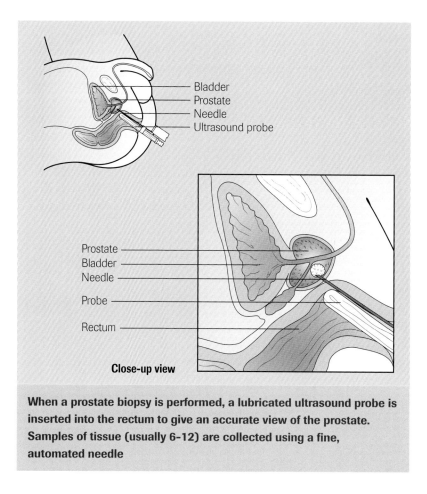

Bladder
Prostate
Needle
Ultrasound probe

Prostate
Bladder
Needle
Probe
Rectum

Close-up view

When a prostate biopsy is performed, a lubricated ultrasound probe is inserted into the rectum to give an accurate view of the prostate. Samples of tissue (usually 6–12) are collected using a fine, automated needle

a picture of the prostate that can then be seen on a screen. Ultrasound is a relatively simple and safe procedure that is not too uncomfortable, but without a biopsy it cannot be used to tell definitively whether or not cancer is present.

Ultrasound-guided biopsy

This is used to obtain samples of tissue from your prostate that can then be sent to the pathology laboratory for analysis under a microscope. The pathologist can check whether cancer is present and, if it is, grade it. You will probably be recommended for biopsy, an out-patient procedure, on the basis of your PSA level.

Using ultrasound for guidance, a fine, automated needle is inserted into the back passage until it reaches the prostate (see diagram on previous page). The test is not too painful (not much worse than a visit to the dentist), but you may feel a sharp needle prick as 6–12 tissue samples are taken, even if a local anaesthetic has been used. The results should be available within a few days.

You will usually be given antibiotics (tablets or an injection) immediately before the procedure, and you will be told to continue taking the prescribed antibiotic tablets for several days afterwards. For several weeks after the procedure, you may notice blood in your urine, semen and/or bowel motions. This is normal, but if you have any worries, consult your doctor. Urinary infections can occasionally occur as a consequence of the biopsy – if you feel a burning sensation on urination, notice that your urine is cloudy and/or smelly, find that you have to urinate more frequently than normal and/or you develop a temperature and feel generally unwell, contact your doctor. He will probably prescribe more antibiotics.

Bone scans

These are a means of checking whether the cancer has spread (metastasized) around the body. Several hours before you have the scan, a mixture containing radioactive particles (radionuclides) will be injected into your arm. The particles then distribute around your body; their pattern, which shows up on the scanner, can reveal dark areas of abnormal blood flow – a sign that cancer may be present. Don't be concerned about the use of radiation here – the amount is so low that the risk to your health is negligible.

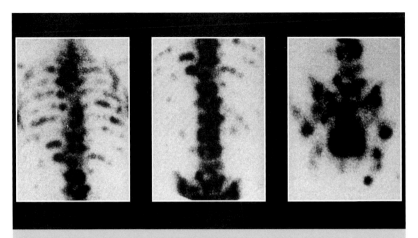

Bone scans from a man with prostate cancer. The dark spots show the presence of secondary tumours

MRI

This is an imaging technique whereby a strong magnetic field and radio signals are used to examine sequential cross-sections of the body. The images that result are highly detailed – the urologist can use them to assess the extent of the cancer in the prostate and to check whether any secondary tumours have formed in other regions. It is not a painful procedure, but some people find being in the scanner a little claustrophobic. If you have any metal implants, such as a pacemaker, it may not be possible to perform an MRI scan. The results should be available within a few days.

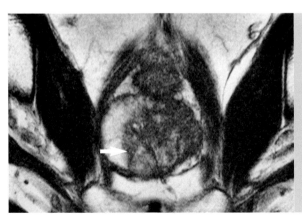

An MRI scan showing cancer (arrowed) in the prostate

27

CT scanning

This is similar to MRI in that the technique produces images of sequential slices through the body, but it uses X-rays to build up the images. CT scanning is not as accurate as MRI, but is much less claustrophobic. Occasionally CT scanning is used to guide biopsy needles to obtain tissue samples from enlarged lymph nodes. It also helps when planning radiotherapy treatment fields.

Partin's tables

Although the tests described above seem very 'high tech' and sophisticated, unfortunately they do not always give a very precise answer to the question 'has the cancer spread beyond the gland?' In fact the so-called 'Partin's tables', which compare the findings at rectal examination, the PSA level and the Gleason score, are still the best way of estimating the risk of spread beyond the prostate capsule.

These tables were developed by Dr Alan Partin, a urologist at Johns Hopkins University Hospital, Baltimore, USA. He has shown that the smaller the cancer feels on rectal examination, and the lower the PSA level and Gleason score, the greater the likelihood that the cancer can be completely removed by surgery. These tables can therefore be useful in helping the doctor and patient decide together on the best treatment option.

Treatment options for prostate cancer that has not spread beyond the gland

The most appropriate treatment for you will depend on several factors:

- how aggressive and advanced your cancer is (the grade and stage)
- your age
- your general health
- your own therapy preferences.

For example, for older men with small tumours and those with other severe illnesses, often the best option is what is known as 'watchful waiting'.

Watchful waiting

When you first hear of this, you may think 'What a cop-out', and media reports of older patients receiving second-rate healthcare may spring to mind. But watchful waiting is not a second-rate option at all – it's often a way of allowing you to retain maximum quality of life.

The chance that a small tumour will cause problems to an older man before the end of his natural life is often relatively small. On balance, the side-effects of the other treatment options would probably cause far greater distress. As the name suggests, although you will not receive treatment, you will have regular check-ups and your urologist will monitor your condition closely.

If you choose the watchful waiting option, you must, for your own peace of mind, be convinced that it is right for you. Despite all the progress made in early diagnosis and treatments, a diagnosis of cancer of any kind is still distressing for the patient and his loved ones. It would be a rare person who, having been told that he has cancer, then manages to put the diagnosis out of his mind. It's all too easy to understand everything and feel confident that you are doing the right thing while you are in the urologist's consulting room, and then a few weeks later start to feel panicked and uneasy that nothing is being done about your condition. Remember that the whole point of watchful waiting is that your quality of life remains good – if you start to worry needlessly, perhaps losing sleep, then your quality of life is suffering. If this happens, pick up the phone or write to your GP or urologist and tell him how you are feeling. You might also find that becoming involved with a support group helps (see page 96).

Radiotherapy

Radiotherapy is appropriate for the younger man whose cancer is confined to the prostate. But it is also suitable for the younger man whose general health precludes major surgery. With this type of treatment, radiation is applied to the affected area – the prostate and surrounding tissues – to destroy the cancer cells. You may be offered one of two types of radiotherapy: external-beam radiotherapy is the most commonly used, but another method, called brachytherapy (see opposite), is also becoming more widely available.

External-beam radiotherapy

As the name suggests, a beam of radiation generated by an external source is directed at your abdomen. This is normally an out-patient procedure, and the most usual pattern of treatment is 20–30 minutes of treatment, 5 days a week for 5–6 weeks.

About 3 months before the radiotherapy, you may be started on hormone therapy (see pages 41 and 42). This shrinks the prostate so that the radiation is more likely to destroy the cancer cells, which are now concentrated in a smaller area.

Recently, a new form of radiotherapy – conformal radiotherapy – has been introduced. This allows better targeting of the cancer and so carries a lower risk of side-effects. Ask your radiotherapist whether it is available in your area.

Possible side-effects and risks. The main side-effects are bladder irritation and a need to urinate more often. Usually these effects are mild, though a very small proportion of men will be severely affected. You may also feel irritation or discomfort around the

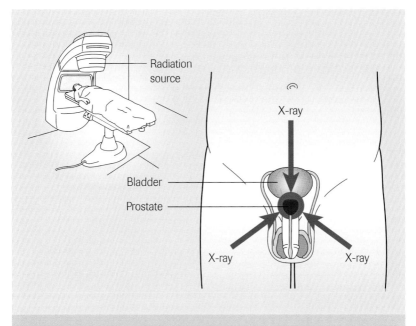

Radiation source

X-ray

Bladder

Prostate

X-ray

X-ray

With external-beam radiotherapy, X-rays are produced by an external radiation source and focused on the prostate from three directions

rectum, and notice some diarrhoea and bleeding; these effects are usually temporary, lasting only for a few weeks, but may persist for a longer time in some men. Very occasionally, the rectal injury is disabling and a colostomy (a bag collecting bowel motions) becomes necessary.

A proportion of men who have undergone radiotherapy will become impotent as a result. This problem tends to develop gradually over 6–12 months, and can often be overcome with the use of treatments such as Viagra (sildenafil).

Brachytherapy

This is a relatively new procedure that has become popular in the USA and, at present, is available in only a few centres in the UK. It involves the implantation of radioactive pellets actually into the prostate, so the radiation is emitted from inside rather than from an external source (as is the case with external-beam radiotherapy). The pellets are left inside the patient where they gradually decay (lose their radioactivity) over the following months.

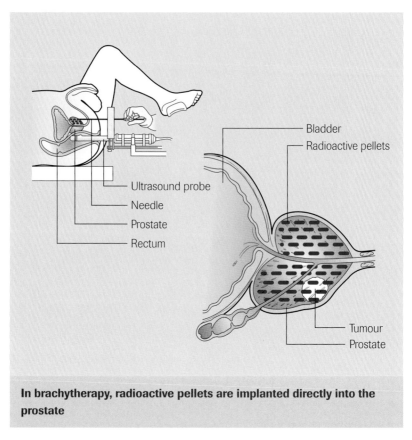

In brachytherapy, radioactive pellets are implanted directly into the prostate

Before the pellets are implanted, the radiotherapist will need to assess your prostate exactly. In order to do so, an ultrasound probe will be inserted into your rectum so that an ultrasound scan can be seen on a computer screen. You will be given either a spinal or general anaesthetic beforehand. The pellets – usually between 60 and 100 – are then put into your prostate using needles inserted through the skin between your scrotum and rectum. A catheter will be inserted to help you pass urine after the operation – this might have to stay in place for a couple of days, but you can normally go home within 24 hours.

Possible side-effects and risks. This is a relatively new technique developed in Seattle. Up to 10 years after treatment, the results appear to be good in terms of keeping the PSA level down and local cancer control. It seems that as the radiation is being targeted

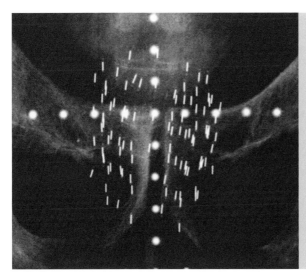

An X-ray showing the radioactive pellets in place in the prostate. The larger dots in the shape of a cross are used to help target the prostate

at the prostate so accurately, urinary problems and rectal damage are probably less common after brachytherapy than after external-beam radiotherapy. Problems with potency, though, are still common. Brachytherapy is not appropriate for men whose cancer has spread beyond the prostate or who have already undergone TURP for BPH (see pages 69–71). Only time will tell just how effective it is.

Radical prostatectomy

A radical prostatectomy is a surgical procedure in which the prostate, seminal vesicles and a sample of some nearby lymph nodes are removed. It's quite a technically difficult operation and, as a result, is carried out only in certain hospitals by surgeons with particular expertise and experience. Because it is a fairly major operation, and major surgery always carries certain risks, a radical prostatectomy is most suitable for otherwise healthy, younger men (generally those under 70) whose cancer appears not to have spread to the distant lymph nodes or bones.

The operation is carried out under a general anaesthetic, and usually takes 1–3 hours; you should expect to stay in hospital for 4–10 days. A cut will be made through your abdomen (or less commonly through the perineum), and your prostate and seminal vesicles will be removed. Samples from the lymph nodes nearest to

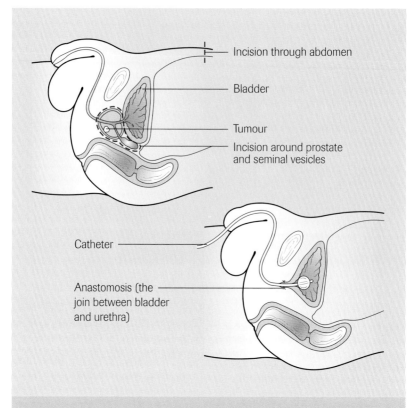

Incision through abdomen

Bladder

Tumour

Incision around prostate and seminal vesicles

Catheter

Anastomosis (the join between bladder and urethra)

In a radical prostatectomy, the entire prostate and seminal vesicles are removed through an incision in the abdomen. Sometimes nearby lymph glands are also removed. The urethra is joined to the bladder and a catheter is inserted to drain urine

your prostate will also be taken to check whether the cancer has spread to these sites. The so-called cavernous nerves, which lie close to the prostate and are important for achieving an erection, will be identified and the surgeon will take particular care not to disturb them (this may not be possible where the cancer has spread very close to the nerves); this is called a nerve-sparing approach. A catheter will be inserted into the penis so that urination can continue while the join (technically called the anastomosis) between the bladder and urethra heals. The catheter will usually have to stay in place for up to a fortnight (so you will often need to go home with it for a week or so).

After a radical prostatectomy

Returning to work

- Possible after 6–8 weeks

- A longer period of absence will be necessary if your job involves heavy lifting

- Your doctor will give you a sick note

Driving

- Do not drive for 2–4 weeks after the operation

Sexual activity

- Do not attempt to have sex for 6–8 weeks

- After this time, you can get back to normal. Orgasm can usually be reached, but there will be no ejaculate and your erection will be weak initially

Drinking

- Try to drink more (non-alcoholic) drinks than you would do normally. The resulting increase in the volume of urine produced can help protect against infection

- You can drink alcohol (but, of course, for your general health, this should be in moderation)

Exercise

- Rest as much as possible for the first 2 weeks

- Avoid any heavy work, such as lifting, carrying or digging, for several months

- Sports and exercise can be resumed after about 1 month, but be guided by how you feel and start off very gently (swimming is a good exercise to begin with)

You'll need to take it easy when you return home from hospital; the usual period of convalescence is 6–8 weeks, but you may still feel tired even after this time. Avoid lifting heavy objects for several months. Some guidelines for what you should and should not do after the operation are shown in the table above.

When further treatment is needed

In between one-tenth to one-third of all men who undergo radical prostatectomy, the cancer will be found to have spread to the margin of the prostate once the pathology report is available. This finding is particularly likely in men whose PSA level is above 10 ng/mL. As a consequence, the operation will sometimes not be 100% successful in these men as the cancer has not been wholly removed from the body. If this is the case for you, your doctor may recommend a 'mop-up' course of radiotherapy or some long-term drug therapy (see pages 41 and 42, anti-androgens). After the operation, your PSA level will be monitored closely – if the operation has been a success, it should remain undetectably low (see page 40, the Pound study). If your PSA starts to rise, you will need further treatment.

Possible side-effects and risks

A radical prostatectomy is major surgery and as such has side-effects that you should consider when deciding whether this is the appropriate course of action for you. For men who may have wanted children, infertility from the surgery needs to be talked through thoroughly with their doctor and partner. Sperm banking is one option that could be considered.

Some men also experience a degree of temporary urinary incontinence after the operation. For most, incontinence is mild – a leakage of a small amount of urine on, for example, coughing. A very small proportion of men have severe incontinence requiring further treatment, but very few have a permanent problem, other than having to wear a small pad for security.

Impotence (difficulty achieving an erection) is another side-effect and affects many men who have undergone a radical prostatectomy. The risk is reduced where a surgeon uses a nerve-sparing approach but, even so, potency cannot be guaranteed. Although impotence can usually be treated quite effectively, the surgeon should discuss this with you in detail prior to surgery, and you should discuss it with your partner.

Internal scarring from the operation is a further potential complication. It may mean that you will have to undergo a dilatation (stretch) of the join between the bladder and urethra; this is usually curative, but sometimes has to be repeated.

On the positive side, for men who have BPH as well as prostate cancer, radical prostatectomy can potentially offer a 'double cure' as the prostate, the source of the BPH symptoms, is removed.

The risks associated with radical prostatectomy are those that generally attach to major surgery – blood loss or blood clots, adverse reaction to the general anaesthetic, and infection. In the best hands, fewer than 1 in 1000 men having the operation will die as a result.

Your chance of side-effects and the likely success of the operation are governed largely by the expertise of your urologist. If you are offered this operation, you should ask your urologist a number of questions.

- How many radical prostatectomies have you performed (more than 100 is a respectable number) and how many in the last year?
- What were the results of these operations, in terms of removing the cancer and of the proportion of patients who were free from the major side-effects of impotence and incontinence?
- Will you be performing my surgery personally?
- Will you be there to help if I have postoperative problems?
- When will the pathology report be available?

Surgery or radiotherapy?

Ultimately, when you have weighed up the pros and cons with your urologist, the choice will be yours. The risks associated with radical prostatectomy or radiotherapy and a summary of the pros and cons of each are shown in the tables below and overleaf.

Risks associated with radical prostatectomy and radiotherapy			
	Men who die as a result	Men who become impotent as a result	Men who suffer mild to severe incontinence
External-beam radiotherapy	Less than 0.1%	30–50%	1–2%
Brachytherapy	Less than 0.1%	30–50%	2%
Radical prostatectomy	0.6%	30–70%	2–15%

The pros and cons of radical prostatectomy versus radiotherapy

Radical prostatectomy

Pros

- Offers a cure for tumours confined to the prostate
- Allows the doctor to stage your tumour accurately
- Coexisting BPH is treated
- Your PSA level should become undetectably low
- You are likely to feel reassured about your condition after the operation
- Monitoring for cancer reappearance is easy
- Radiotherapy can be given afterwards if the cancer returns

Cons

- Major surgery
- Small risk of severe bleeding associated with operation
- Success/side-effects depend on the skill of the urologist
- Possible side-effects (see text)

Radiotherapy/brachytherapy

Pros

- Offers a potential cure
- Avoids prolonged catheterization and surgery
- Given on an out-patient or short-stay basis
- Hormone therapy can increase the chance of success

Cons

- Treatment is prolonged (6 weeks in external-beam radiotherapy)
- It is relatively difficult to assess whether the treatment has been successful
- Accurate staging is not possible
- Coexisting BPH is untreated
- You may feel more concerned about the possible chance of success afterwards
- Your PSA level may not drop to very low levels
- Repeat radiation treatment is not possible
- Surgery after radiotherapy carries greater risks and is only suitable for selected cases
- Possible side-effects (see text)

How do I make the choice?

Until the results of ongoing studies are available, it will not be known for certain which is the best treatment for localized prostate cancer. Until then, there will be a choice of treatments which the patient must decide for himself. Critical to this choice is the confidence that you feel in your doctor, so it is important to find a good specialist and weigh up the pros and cons with him, before deciding for yourself which treatment is right for you.

The long-term picture

Long-term studies provide information on the prospects of men who have undergone these procedures. While many men want this kind of information, it is important *not* to take the figures given here too much to heart without discussing your own individual circumstances with your urologist. Progress in medicine means that patients' long-term prospects are improving all the time, and in due course the results of ongoing trials will resolve many controversies.

Watchful waiting

The likelihood that your cancer will spread depends, as we have already said, on the nature of your cancer (that is, how aggressive it is). For men whose cancer has a low Gleason score, the 10-year survival rate is 87% (this means that, after 10 years, 87 men in 100 will not have died from prostate cancer; conversely, 13 men in 100 will have died from their prostate cancer). With more aggressive cancers (those with higher Gleason scores), the survival rate drops considerably (the 10-year survival rate for men with poorly differentiated tumours has been put at 26%).

Radical prostatectomy

More than 80% of men who have this operation are alive 10 years afterwards, and 60% are still alive at 15 years. A Scandinavian study has just been reported comparing the long-term outcomes of men who have watchful waiting with those who have radical prostatectomy. These results suggest that radical prostatectomy is the treatment option most likely to offer a complete cure for younger men, as it physically removes both the cancer and the entire prostate from the body, making recurrence much less likely.

Results from a very recent study by Pound and colleagues confirm that 82% of men undergoing this procedure at Johns Hopkins Hospital in Baltimore (USA) were free of recurrence at 15 years (as determined by PSA measurement). The study also offers some comfort to the man whose PSA level rises years after the operation. As we have already said, after a radical prostatectomy, your PSA level drops to an undetectable level, and a re-emerging PSA result can signal cancer recurrence. The data from the study in question indicate that, though this is the case, the cancer spreads in only around one-third of men with elevated PSA. Furthermore, unless a man had a particularly aggressive cancer (in which case his PSA level would tend to rise relatively quickly after the operation), the spreading cancer would not become life-threatening for several years, and would likely be amenable to treatment by radiotherapy or LHRH analogues (see page 41).

Radiotherapy
At best, the survival rates with radiotherapy are comparable to those associated with radical prostatectomy. Several published studies have put the 15-year survival rates at 40–60% (that is, between 40 and 60 men in 100 will still be alive after 15 years). Recent data suggest that the use of luteinizing hormone releasing hormone (LHRH) injections or anti-androgens to shrink the prostate ahead of radiotherapy can increase the chance that treatment will be successful (see pages 41 and 42). The risk of serious side-effects with radiotherapy is decreasing as improved technology means that the cancer-destroying rays can be targeted more accurately at the cancer. Brachytherapy proponents also report improving results as techniques and patient selection are enhanced. However, problems with potency are still frequently encountered after radiotherapy and in fact are more common when this treatment is combined with hormone therapy.

If prostate cancer has spread or recurs after treatment

Locally advanced disease

If your cancer has spread outside your prostate, but has not yet spread to the lymph nodes close by or to more distant locations, it is described as being 'locally advanced'. (In the TNM staging system, this state is known as T_3–N_0–M_0.) Treatment options are:

- watchful waiting (for older, less fit men, as before)
- hormone therapy
- intermittent hormone therapy
- hormone therapy followed by radical prostatectomy
- hormone therapy followed by radiotherapy
- anti-androgen monotherapy.

Watchful waiting

The rationale behind adopting this approach has been outlined earlier (see pages 29–30). However, it is important to realize that at this stage, because the cancer is more advanced, it is likely to cause symptoms and become life-threatening more quickly than a low-grade cancer that is still confined to the prostate.

Hormone therapy

This is sometimes called 'cytoreduction', and has been touched on in the previous section. There are usually two components:

- luteinizing hormone releasing hormone (LHRH) analogues; LHRH is a naturally occurring hormone, and the 'analogue' part of the name means that it is a synthetic form that has a structure similar to the natural form
- anti-androgens, which block the action of testosterone in the body.

Testosterone, an androgen or male hormone, is produced in the testicles and has the effect of stimulating cancer growth. The aim of hormone therapy is to reduce the effect of testosterone by switching off testosterone production (the LHRH analogues) and/or by dampening its effects on the cancer (the anti-androgens). The overall effect is that the tumour size is reduced and the progression of the tumour is delayed (hormone therapy does not offer a complete cure, however).

Usually, implants containing a LHRH analogue are inserted by injection at either monthly or 3-monthly intervals. Your body may react to the first injection by initially increasing the amount of testosterone it makes – this is the so-called 'flare' effect. To counter this, you'll probably be given anti-androgens to take before and at the beginning of treatment with the LHRH analogue.

Possible side-effects. As a consequence of stopping the production of testosterone, men receiving a LHRH analogue lose their sex drive and are unable to achieve an erection. This is gradually reversed if the drug is stopped. Some men also experience hot flushes – these may be eased by low doses (50 mg/day) of Cyprostat (cyproterone acetate).

Anti-androgens may cause mild stomach upsets and diarrhoea. Rarely, they can have a deleterious effect on your liver (so you will need regular blood tests while you are taking these tablets).

How effective is hormone therapy? Hormone therapy alone reduces the tumour size and slows the cancer progression in around 80% of men with locally advanced disease. It does not destroy all the cancer cells, so the cancer is not cured, but its progression is significantly delayed.

Intermittent hormone therapy

This is a newer approach to hormone therapy. An LHRH analogue is given for about 36 weeks and is then discontinued (providing the PSA level has dropped down to a normal value). When the PSA level returns to a predetermined level, the hormone treatment is started again. Some doctors believe that this might make the cancer cells susceptible to the drug for longer than they would be if treatment was continued without a break. Studies looking at the long-term safety and effectiveness of this approach are under way but for the moment it is still experimental.

Hormone therapy followed by radical prostatectomy
Some doctors believe that shrinking the tumour with hormone therapy before carrying out a radical prostatectomy increases the chance of removing all the cancer. This approach is being tested in long-term studies. The latest data suggest, however, that there are no concrete, long-term advantages to having hormone treatment before surgery, so this approach is not generally recommended.

Hormone therapy followed by radiotherapy
Again, studies are being carried out to see whether hormone treatment before radiotherapy gives better results than radiotherapy alone. In this case, the results are encouraging, suggesting that the hormone treatment does indeed offer a benefit in terms of curing, or at least delaying, the progress of disease. This is probably because the shrunken tumour is more susceptible to the anti-cancer effects of ionizing radiation.

Anti-androgen monotherapy
There is now scientific evidence that an anti-androgen drug alone (i.e. monotherapy) can also help to slow the progress of advanced cancer, particularly when bone metastases are not present. The advantage of this approach is that anti-androgens have less effect on sex drive and are less likely to cause impotence than the injectable LHRH analogues. Breast tenderness and enlargement can occur, but though these side-effects can be troublesome, they usually disappear if treatment is stopped. Liver function is only rarely disturbed by agents such as Casodex (bicalutamide), but blood testing should be performed regularly to exclude this.

Metastatic disease

Once cancer has spread to the lymph nodes and to distant sites, such as the bones, it is referred to as metastatic disease (the metastases are the secondary growths that occur at the distant site). This is an advanced form of cancer, and one that is associated with a relatively poor outlook – around 70% of men affected will have died from their cancer within 5 years.

Treatment options are available to men with this stage of cancer, however, and can delay progression of the disease and death for several years. The treatments are:

- orchidectomy (removal of both testicles)
- hormone therapy with LHRH analogues
- 'maximal androgen blockade', which is hormone therapy with a combination of LHRH analogue and anti-androgen.

Orchidectomy

This is a surgical procedure in which the testicles are removed. The reasoning behind this is that, as testosterone is produced in the testicles, their removal stops its production altogether. Most men (70–80%) respond positively to this treatment, with the progression of their cancer slowing markedly for around 18 months.

The operation is straightforward, and is performed under a local or general anaesthetic in around 30 minutes. In selected patients, silicone testicular prostheses may be inserted to improve the cosmetic result. The scrotal sac is opened and the testicles are snipped out. You may be allowed out of hospital on the same day, although often your surgeon will want you to stay in overnight to check for bruising. You must take things easy for a week or two, and you should also take regular baths or showers to keep the wound clean. Afterwards, the scrotum will look somewhat shrivelled and empty, unless prostheses have been used.

Although the operation appears rather drastic, and some men are concerned about 'castration' and the appearance of their scrotum afterwards, it is a one-off procedure and so avoids the need to take a prolonged course of hormone therapy.

Possible side-effects and risks. As your body will be unable to produce testosterone after the operation, you will lose your sex drive and be unable to achieve an erection. You will also be infertile. These effects are irreversible, so consider the implications fully before consenting to an orchidectomy. Potential complications of the surgery are few, but bruising, blood clots and infections do occur in some men. Hot flushes may result from the hormone changes in your body. You won't become 'feminized' or find that your voice changes, but you may notice that you lose some body hair and may have to shave rather less often. There is also often a change in skin texture.

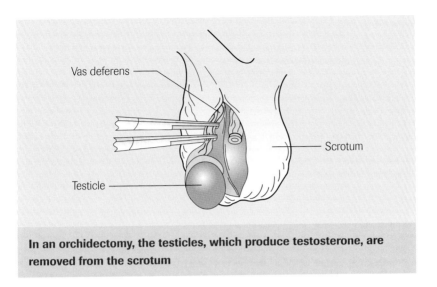

In an orchidectomy, the testicles, which produce testosterone, are removed from the scrotum

Hormone therapy

LHRH analogues (see pages 41 and 42) work by blocking testosterone production, and hence reduce the stimulation of cancer growth. LHRH analogues, such as Zoladex (goserelin), are usually administered in an implant form, with the implant lying just under the skin of your abdomen. They are put in place by means of an injection. The procedure is repeated every month or 3 months. As with orchidectomy, a high proportion of men (more than 80%) respond to this treatment, and the beneficial effects usually last for around 18–36 months. In terms of effectiveness and safety, there is little to choose between hormone therapy and orchidectomy.

Possible side-effects and risks. At first, the LHRH analogue actually increases testosterone production for a few days. Bone pain may increase as a consequence, and urinary symptoms may worsen. There is even a remote risk of the cancer causing pressure on the spinal cord and paralysis. To counter these effects, anti-androgens are usually given for 2 weeks before and then for the first 2–6 weeks of LHRH analogue treatment; these effectively block the effect of testosterone on the cancer.

Maximal androgen blockade

This combines the use of LHRH analogues with long-term anti-androgens. Whether or not this approach is superior to that using

LHRH analogues only or orchidectomy is not entirely clear. Some studies show men respond for a longer length of time with this treatment, while others have failed to show such an effect. Many doctors do have confidence in this approach, though, and feel that it is particularly appropriate for younger, relatively fit men with advanced prostate cancer.

Possible side-effects. As outlined previously, treatment with LHRH analogues results in a loss of sex drive and impotence. Hot flushes can also be a problem but sometimes respond to treatment with Cyprostat (50 mg/day). The other part of the treatment, anti-androgens, may upset your stomach and can sometimes cause diarrhoea. Very occasionally, anti-androgens cause liver problems, so regular blood tests will be performed while you are receiving this treatment to monitor the health of your liver.

Recurrence

Almost inevitably, cancers that initially respond to the above hormonal treatments eventually begin to grow again (see the diagram on the page opposite for an explanation of why this happens). This stage of prostate cancer is often referred to as 'hormone-escaped' disease.

If you reach this stage, your doctor may recommend one of the following treatment options:

- modifying existing hormonal therapy by adding or withdrawing anti-androgen
- cytotoxic chemotherapy (drugs that destroy the cancer cells)
- hormone therapy (this is different from that discussed earlier)
- another form of treatment that aims to prevent substances in the body from stimulating further growth of the cancer.

Cytotoxic chemotherapy

This is one option, but the drugs used can have unpleasant side-effects, such as sickness and hair loss. An increasing number of chemotherapy drugs are now available, so if your doctor discusses this with you, ask what side-effects you might expect and whether it is possible to counter them effectively. Oncologists rather than urologists are experts in this area.

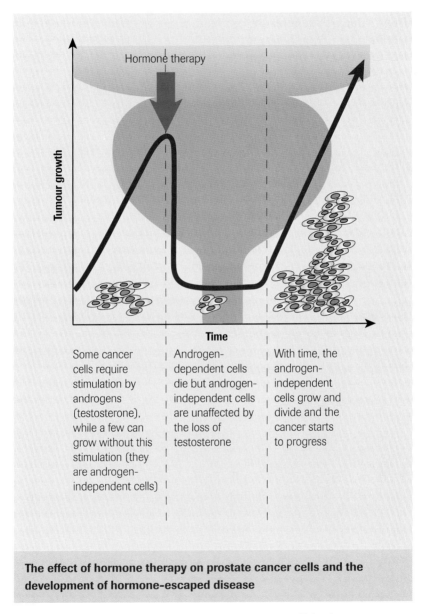

The effect of hormone therapy on prostate cancer cells and the development of hormone-escaped disease

So what is the point of these drugs? It is possible that chemotherapy might give you an extra few months or even years, and if the side-effects are minimal or can be overcome, you might feel that this option is worthwhile. Another point is that new drugs, such as taxotere, are on the horizon that may offer better survival rates, and these may be available quite soon – your urologist and the oncologist he works with will be able to discuss the latest treatments with you.

Hormone treatment

Oestrogens, female hormones, may offer some benefit at this stage of your disease. They appear to be able to reduce stimulation of cancer growth and they may also damage the cancer cells directly. The reason that oestrogens are not used in earlier disease is that they can have some potentially serious side-effects, such as nausea, blood clots and other cardiovascular complications, such as heart attacks or even strokes. Many doctors advise that you take a low dose (75 mg) of aspirin if you take oestrogen-based drugs to help overcome the potential cardiovascular side-effects. A Chinese herbal preparation known as PC-Spes was popular with some patients. It contains plant oestrogens (and is rather expensive), but there is very little scientific evidence available yet to support its effectiveness or to show that it's safe. Indeed, recently it was withdrawn from sale after it was shown that there were serious problems with impurities and contamination.

Other treatments

There are a number of what are called 'growth factors' in the body that stimulate the progression of prostate cancer. Blocking the action of these growth factors should block their stimulatory effects on the cancer. However, the drugs that are being developed with this aim are very new, and are still under investigation. Angiogenesis inhibitors have already been mentioned (see page 10). Again though, if and when you reach this stage, knowledge of the effects of these drugs may be such that your doctor is able to prescribe them for you.

Palliative care

This aims to provide you with support to make you feel comfortable in the final stages of the illness. Over recent years, considerable progress has been made in this area, and medical opinion now holds that no patient needs to feel the pain or discomfort that was characteristic of the last stages of cancer in bygone years. If your cancer progresses to this stage, you will usually be assigned a palliative care team – specialist doctors and nurses who have considerable expertise and experience in this area. You will have opportunities to talk to members of the team about your care, and you should discuss any specific areas that are troubling you, no matter how trivial you think they may appear.

Patients with very advanced prostate cancer tend to experience bone pain, and you will be given strong and effective painkillers to help overcome this. In addition, you might have radiotherapy (either as a short course or a one-off). Another effective method of alleviating bone pain is with injections of a radioactive substance known as strontium. If you are offered radiotherapy, make sure that you know whether it is likely to result in other side-effects, such as nausea and vomiting, so that you can weigh up the advantages and disadvantages in the light of all the facts and your own personal circumstances.

Prostate cancer – the future

The prospects for significant progress in prostate cancer in the near future are good. We can hopefully look forward to effective prevention, earlier diagnosis, better staging, and more effective and less toxic therapy. A number of current research endeavours may well translate into improved quality of life and improved survival prospects for those affected by prostate cancer.

Chemoprevention

In the future, it may be possible to prevent prostate cancer. Already there is some evidence that both vitamin E and selenium may have a preventative effect (see page 12). The benefits of the 5α-reductase inhibitor Proscar (finasteride) are also currently being assessed in a large trial, and several other agents appear to show promise but require further research to ensure their safety and effectiveness.

Better diagnosis

Earlier detection, while the disease is still curable, is already a reality as a result of PSA testing. In the future, new tests or variations of existing tests will continue to improve the ability of doctors and surgeons to distinguish early prostate cancer from BPH. It also seems likely that it will soon be possible to predict the behaviour of individual prostate cancers more accurately, which will make it easier for patients and their doctors to decide which is the best treatment option.

New treatments
Laparoscopic prostatectomy
Surgeons in France, the USA and the UK have recently performed radical prostatectomy laparoscopically, using telescopes and four small incisions. This technique has much promise for the future and may soon be robotically assisted. At present, however, it is still under development and available in only a few centres.

Cryotherapy

This technique uses freezing to destroy the prostatic tissue. An ultrasound probe in the rectum enables the position of the prostate to be seen on a computer screen. Eight 'cryogenic' probes are then inserted into the prostate, and liquid nitrogen is circulated to reduce the temperature to around –180°C. At this temperature, the tissue surrounding the probes is destroyed. The urethra is protected by circulating warm water through a catheter. Some studies have reported survival rates similar to those achieved with radical prostatectomy, but others described rectal and urethral damage, and no long-term randomized, controlled trials to compare cryotherapy with established treatments have yet been carried out.

High-intensity focused ultrasound (HIFU)

This new technology allows ultrasound waves to be focused on prostate cancer cells. It can be used to treat both newly diagnosed cancers and recurrences after radiotherapy. Initial results look encouraging, but more work needs to be done.

Drug treatments

As new anti-androgens are developed, it is likely that they will be used at earlier stages of the disease when the cancer cells are more sensitive to the blocking of the action of testosterone.

Research is also being carried out into drugs that inhibit the growth factors that have been shown to be necessary for the development and progression of prostate cancer. These drugs also offer the possibility of fewer side-effects and greater effectiveness.

Immunotherapy

Work on harnessing the immune system to counter prostate cancer may make it possible to vaccinate men at high risk of the disease.

Gene therapy

Spectacular advances in molecular biology have made the prospect of gene therapy a reality. In the not too distant future, it may be possible to 'turn off' the oncogenes that induce cancer and 'turn on' the protective tumour suppressor genes. New therapies will also be developed that selectively destroy prostate cancer by activating the in-built cell suicide system known as 'apoptosis'.

Frequently asked questions about prostate cancer

Prostate Research Campaign UK thanks Clive Turner, a patient who has had radical prostate surgery himself and an experienced counsellor of hundreds of men with prostate cancer, for writing this section. The questions he answers here reflect his own views and the many common concerns of those men who approach him for advice.

Is there much on the internet about prostate cancer? Yes, heaps, and a lot of it unvalidated, and very 'fringe' in nature, but you can certainly learn a good deal if you are selective in your reading. But Prostate Research Campaign UK (www.prostate-research.org.uk) and other charities have websites, leaflets and other publications available (see pages 96 and 97) which are more factual and much less alarming.

How reliable is the PSA test? It is not a perfect test, but it is the best we have at present, and is considered extremely useful by most urologists, especially if it is expertly evaluated, and taken together with a DRE. Yes, there are false PSA readings, and they can alarm needlessly, but PSA tests undoubtedly save lives, and the Department of Health has recently sanctioned PSA tests in informed men aged 50–70. The test can assist in telling the difference between cancerous and benign conditions of the prostate (the latter being inconvenient, but not life-threatening).

If cancer is diagnosed, should I have radiotherapy, surgery, or should I 'watch and wait'? That depends on many factors, including your location, age, the results of biopsies, PSA levels, and your general health. And expert opinions do differ, but get them anyway, and weigh them up very carefully before making any decision.

Radiation therapy (and there are various kinds, including brachytherapy) can be very successful for some patients, meaning the tumour cells are killed off while the prostate is kept intact (though there are sometimes unpleasant side-effects, such as rectal inflammation, while the therapy is undertaken and thereafter). But for those whose tumours reappear later, even after some years, the possibility of successful surgery then is frankly quite low.

Bear in mind that repeated radiation is not possible in the long term, and it must be pointed out that ultimate success with radiation therapy is currently not much over 50–70%, even with improved techniques. By contrast, with a radical prostatectomy, although radical by definition, the success rate in removing tumour and preventing recurrence is commonly over 80%. If you feel lucky or confident about your chances, then radiation therapy may well be for you, but think about it and weigh up the options carefully.

If you decide to watch and wait, make sure you have regular check-ups to see if the situation is changing, and if so, to what extent. If cancer is present, it can stay dormant, grow slowly or accelerate rapidly, for reasons that are not yet fully understood.

Why are certain patients ineligible for brachytherapy?
Brachytherapy is most suitable for patients with smaller, lower risk cancers and for men who have small or medium-sized prostates. If TURP has been performed previously, the radioactive seeds cannot be sited correctly in the gland. Pre-treatment with prostate-shrinking drugs such as LHRH analogues can sometimes make brachytherapy suitable for men with large glands.

What are the commonest side-effects of radiotherapy? During treatment you will often feel tired, urinate frequently and have rectal irritation. In a small proportion of patients, the rectal symptoms persist and are associated with rectal bleeding.

Consultants ordinarily recommend a biopsy, or even more than one, to see what degree of cancer may be present if the PSA level is raised above the norm (greater than 4 ng/mL). I am told this can be very painful and unpleasant. Is this true, and why is it necessary? Biopsies are not exactly thrilling or agreeable to experience; they can be very uncomfortable or, at worst, rather painful. They can also cause rectal bleeding and blood in the ejaculate, but this has been likened to having a nosebleed, and it will stop. Nowadays, doctors taking biopsies from the prostate, via the rectum, will often use a local anaesthetic, especially if you ask for one.

The results of the biopsy will indicate whether tumours are present, although the tests are not infallible, and they can give negative readings if they happen to miss a tumour altogether. And pathologists who examine prostates that have been removed by surgeons commonly find much more cancer present than the biopsies had indicated, given that some evidence of tumour had originally been revealed.

And again, consultants sometimes want you to have a bone scan, CT scan or MRI before they will deliberate on the best course of treatment. Why is this? Because this may reveal whether any cancer has spread to other parts of the body, having 'escaped' from the prostate gland. If this has happened, urologists will avoid surgery, and may well recommend radiation and/or hormone therapy in such a circumstance. Remember, though, that these tests do not give a perfect answer to the question 'Has the cancer spread?'

So, if I go for surgery, is the operation painful? Not really, because any pain is expertly controlled. This can be achieved, for example, through the use of epidural anaesthetics and of drugs given to you postoperatively.

Is there much loss of blood? No, not normally. Only a small proportion (about 10%) of patients undergoing radical prostatectomy nowadays require a blood transfusion, possibly about two pints – not a particularly significant quantity.

Do I need to have some of my own blood taken beforehand? No, unless it will buy you peace of mind, but if there are no exceptional circumstances there is no need. Use of your own (autologous) blood is more common in the USA, where there is possibly a higher risk of infection from regular blood transfusion. It is not advised in the UK.

While on the subject of blood, I have heard that you see traces of blood in the urine after the operation. Is this true and why is it? It is true, but normally it is only a trace, and just while the catheter is draining urine immediately after the operation, or perhaps for a while longer while the re-routed 'plumbing' inside is healing. It normally clears after a week or two at most. Drinking extra fluids is helpful, as is taking laxatives, wholewheat cereal, prune juice and fruit to keep the bowels regular.

Is there any risk that I will die during or shortly after the operation? There is always such a risk (around 1 in 1000), but I personally have yet to hear of one example. Don't be afraid to ask your surgeon what his own mortality rate is.

What about unsightly scars as a result of the operation? This need be the least of your concerns. To gain access to the prostate, many surgeons perform an 8–10 cm lateral or vertical incision above the pubic bone, with a small drain hole beside it. Clips are more commonly used than stitches these days, and the healing process is quick. Indeed after a few months the scar is almost, but not quite, invisible. Recently laparoscopic radical prostatectomy has been performed, and results in smaller scars, but a longer operation time. This procedure is still in development.

How long will I be in hospital? Between 4 and 7 days, often including a 12–24-hour period in a progressive care ward where you will be monitored for bleeding, signs of respiratory infection, or any heart rate instability. About a fortnight after the operation, your catheter will be removed and you will be watched closely for 24 hours to make sure the new 'plumbing' is in order (for example, your fluid intake will be checked against your urine output).

When will I know if the surgeon has successfully excised the cancer? He will tell you what he thinks within 24 hours, but he has to wait for a few days for the laboratory report on the removed prostate to be sure what has been achieved. If the report is such that some cells are thought to have escaped from the prostate into the surrounding tissue, then the surgeon may recommend some 'mop-up' radiation, which is usually very successful. The radiation therapy doesn't have that much to do compared with clearing the whole prostate of cancer (in contrast to what is necessary if surgery isn't performed). Side-effects are not usually too troublesome, although some rectal irritation and minor bleeding may occur.

Will the PSA have dropped out of sight after the operation? Yes, it should have dropped to about 0.6 ng/mL or thereabouts immediately after the operation, and then gradually reduce further to an ideal of below 0.1 where, in successful cases, it will remain for the rest of your life. But remember to have it checked every 3 months for at least a year, and at the same laboratory too, otherwise you may get a variation in results that could alarm you. In other words, one laboratory may have machines that only read as low as 0.5, whereas another might read down to 0.1, or even 0.01. In essence the result, as far as you are concerned, is the same.

How many years do I have to have these tests? The recommended time frame is 5 years or longer for any cancer to be declared truly gone, but after 3 years with no PSA rise, you can assume your chances of a normal life expectancy are excellent. However, it is still worth having your PSA checked annually as late recurrences can occur.

Are there any special things I need to remember when I am in hospital? Yes. Don't encourage too many visitors; don't worry about breaking wind (nurses love wind because it shows things are beginning to sort themselves out in the bowel, which will have been a bit disturbed during the operation); don't eat too heavy a diet because you don't want to get constipated through lack of exercise and too many heavy meals; drink as much as you can – at least 8 pints of water or soft drinks, like cranberry juice, every day for a couple of weeks if you can stand that (it helps to flush the system through after your internal plumbing has been re-routed); and, most importantly, just look forward to the new future that the surgeon will have given you.

Is it true that my penis will be shorter after the operation? Well, yes, some men have noticed a detectable change in length, but not circumference, when the penis is at rest once everything has settled down. But it's somewhat relative. It rather depends upon how well endowed (as the expression goes) you were to begin with. If there is a noticeable difference, it is very slight. It is because the newly organized and re-routed urethra has been necessarily shortened and therefore had the effect of 'pulling back' the penis into the body just a little. After a few months, the urethra will stretch to accommodate most of the change. On erection, the difference is usually of little or no consequence.

I have heard that after the operation my scrotum and possibly my penis will be very badly swollen and look severely bruised. What will they have done to them and why is this? This is seldom mentioned before the operation because it is of no long-term significance, but yes, there can be some rather alarming-looking swelling – more often associated with the scrotum, which can occasionally swell to the size of a small orange – but it subsides quite quickly, doesn't hurt, and is neither damaging nor even particularly inconvenient or uncomfortable. The penis can appear a bit bruised also, and this has to do with inevitable disturbance (during the operation) of the blood vessels and nerve endings serving the scrotum. But it really is a very short-term problem and is soon history.

Do I need any special nursing care when I first go home? Not normally, though you may need some help getting up from deep armchairs, or getting into and out of bed during the first few days at home. And it is advisable to wear loose clothes like tracksuit bottoms because your lower tummy will be a bit swollen, and getting zips done up can be a problem for a while. Also you need a spare urine collection leg bag, which the hospital can give you, or you can buy them easily from chemists. You need to keep yourself scrupulously clean to reduce the risks of any infection while the catheter is still in place.

Is it painful to have the catheter removed? Not normally, because catheters are much slimmer these days. Usually it only takes a moment and it's gone, but they can occasionally get a little stuck because of a tight fit – which in fact is a good thing in some respects. If this does happen, a doctor will help with the removal, and frankly that can be somewhat eye-watering in effect unless they give you a sedative at the time. But a modern catheter getting severely stuck is unusual, and you would have to be unlucky to experience it.

Will I feel tired and washed out after the operation? Yes, you will, and this is a normal protective mechanism to allow healing. Some men feel a tremendous loss of energy, and have days when they think they will never regain their original verve, but gradually the energy level returns and the postoperative tiredness and lassitude soon become forgotten.

How long should I be off work? Between 6 and 8 weeks is recommended, although reading, telephone calls, and stress-free activity are all fine. Every single patient with whom I have spoken who has returned to work a bit early has really regretted it, and his recovery has taken longer. Remember, nobody is indispensable, and it will probably do your colleagues the world of good to shoulder some of your responsibilities while you are away! Even if you are retired, take it easy, and handle one day at a time. You can't really drive comfortably for a month, anyway, so get somebody to drive you!

Can I exercise after the operation? Yes, but listen to your body; it will tell you how much is sensible and when to rest. But avoid heavy lifting, such as weight training.

Will I lose my continence control? Not unless you are very unlucky. Most patients now recover control almost as soon as the catheter is taken away, but it is true that for some it can take a few hours, a few days, a few weeks, and even a few months, and you might need to wear some padding for a while if leakage is a bit of a problem. As explained earlier, many surgeons ask you to stay in hospital overnight after the removal of the catheter, measuring fluid intake and outflow to see that the plumbing is working as it should and that there are no internal leaks. To some extent, regaining continence control depends upon individual muscle tone (and you will be taught exercises to strengthen the pelvic muscles), the skill of the surgeon who will have done all he can to spare the nerves that affect continence, and a certain amount of incalculable individual luck. The good news is that things almost always dry up sooner rather than later, and you should have a urine stream like when you were a teenager. If the urinary stream does deteriorate, alert your urologist. You may be developing a bladder neck contracture, which requires gentle stretching under light anaesthetic.

Is sexual dysfunction a problem? Yes, for nearly everyone, whatever they claim. However, some ability and sensation, albeit with a dry orgasm (because the seminal vesicles have been removed as part of the operation) can return after a few months, or sooner for a few lucky ones. Normal penetrative sex is a problem because however careful the surgeon was to avoid damaging the nerves during the operation, achieving a sustainable firm erection is more difficult for most patients, although some men say they can manage reasonably satisfactorily. Having a successful radical prostatectomy is unquestionably a trade-off because if the alternative is to die of prostate cancer, then it has to be remembered that so far as we know there is not a great deal of sex in the graveyard. (Although my local vicar, who incidentally has undergone a radical prostatectomy, told me that there is rather too much in his!)

Sexual dysfunction is also quite common after radiotherapy.

Are there things I can do to help me get back my erections? Yes, there are silicone implants (for those who wish to afford them privately), and these work rather like a bendy toy, in the sense that you bend it up when you want that, and down when you don't. It has to be said, however, that some men have complained that when swimming or playing sports, they can occasionally appear to have a half erection in place, which can be understandably embarrassing. Inflatable penile prostheses produce a more life-like result, but are considerably more expensive and also prone to malfunction.

There are penile injections of prostaglandin which are uncomfortable but not too painful, and provide an almost immediate erection which lasts well, but some men instinctively find it difficult to give themselves such injections.

Vacuum pumps can also help. After an erection has been achieved, it is held in place by a rubber ring slipped over the base of

59

the penis. Although effective, some find such a device scarcely conducive to spontaneity.

Penile suppositories of prostaglandin (known as MUSE) are available, but are quite expensive. They do work, though, and are favoured by some patients.

And now, of course, there is Viagra (sildenafil). Some surgeons are suggesting it be tried about 3–4 months after the operation. But it doesn't seem to work so well until some 6–9 months or so have passed. And then for those with no contraindicated medical history, such as angina or a recent heart attack, Viagra can be very effective, especially at the higher dose of 100 mg. If the drug is used with common sense, many patients have reported results little short of amazing, with very few side-effects of consequence. Perhaps a little face flushing or a headache, but after about an hour, sex is possible with a good erection, providing there is physical stimulus. It doesn't work as the other methods do. It needs sexual stimulus, and then it can often provide repeated satisfaction over a period of some 12 hours. The tablets should not be taken more than once in a 24-hour period, and you should never mix Viagra with nitrates (used to treat angina). Amyl nitrite, also known as 'poppers', is popular with the gay community, but this should *never* be used along with Viagra. Such a practice could prove highly dangerous. Viagra works by relaxing the blood vessels in the penis so allowing the blood to flow there more freely. It is a drug that can now be prescribed on the NHS for prostate cancer sufferers or diabetic men. Don't buy Viagra through the internet.

Other drugs such as Uprima (apomorphine) can be helpful. Successors to Viagra, known as Cialis (tadalafil) and vardenafil, are in the pipeline and may act more quickly and stay effective for longer.

How will my partner be affected? Nobody can 'catch' prostate cancer from you, but your partner will certainly be affected if impotence is the result. Frank discussion is vital before and after the operation, particularly if you go for a radical prostatectomy, and that partner must understand the implications along with you.

Should I tell my family and friends I have, or have had, a cancer? It's up to you of course, but why should there be a need for secrecy and shame, and why not become an advocate for regular check-ups and possibly save a life in the process? This is particularly true if you have sons or brothers who have yet to reach their 40s and 50s when a check-up would be wise, unless by then medical science has beaten this disease completely.

Will the cancer come back? Well, yes, this has been known, with any of the treatments, but is less likely after skilled surgery, followed by mop-up radiation in some cases, and current success rates are reassuringly high. If the PSA does start to rise, treatment with the anti-androgen Casodex (bicalutamide) has been shown to halve the risk of progression.

Was there anything I could have done to prevent the cancer in the first place? Not really, because nobody knows for certain why anyone is affected by it. There are plenty of theories. Some say it is all to do with diet (ranging from eating too much red meat, to eating a lot of ice cream); others believe it is a genetic disease (and there is much research going on in that direction); yet others say it is connected with a multifarious and largely unidentifiable mix of factors, including having had a vasectomy. Nobody has a monopoly of wisdom on the subject. The latest research has found that men who carry a damaged version of a mutant gene are four to five times more likely to suffer from prostate cancer than those who do not have this faulty gene. It's a case of 'watch this space'.

And what about the future in terms of treatments? There is much research going on that may one day find a solution for prostate cancer, through a vaccine, gene therapy or a more certain cure without losing the gland, but we are presently years away from this happy circumstance. And, inevitably, more research money is needed – see page 106!

Symptoms, diagnosis and treatment of BPH

Nearly half (43%) of men over the age of 65 have either urinary symptoms or a reduced urinary flow due to benign prostatic hyperplasia (BPH). BPH is characterized by the benign (non-cancerous) overgrowth of prostate cells, with the effect that the middle portion of the prostate progressively enlarges. The result is that the part of the urethra that is surrounded by the prostate becomes constricted, so the urinary flow is reduced and the man finds that his urine stream becomes weaker and it is more difficult to empty his bladder.

In response to the increasing obstruction, the bladder's walls, which are muscular, thicken and become stronger. Consequently, the pressure inside the bladder needed to produce urinary flow has to increase to overcome the effect of the obstruction, and this high pressure causes pouches or 'diverticula' to form. Less commonly, the raised pressure results in what is known as back pressure on the kidneys, causing kidney problems. If BPH is not treated, either chronic urinary retention (characterized by a massively distended bladder) or acute urinary retention (the sudden and painful inability to pass any urine) may develop. In either situation, hospital admission, catheterization and eventually prostate surgery are usually required.

Why do some men suffer more than others?

Recent work has clarified the risk factors linked to an increased likelihood of developing complications of BPH. The larger the prostate (as assessed by digital rectal examination, DRE), the greater the risk. Similarly, the risk is increased among those with a PSA level above 1.3 ng/mL. Also more likely to develop complications are men whose urine tends to flow slowly and those who have a relatively large amount of urine left in their bladder after attempting to urinate. Although not all men suffer progressive deterioration, in the majority of cases the symptoms gradually become worse over time.

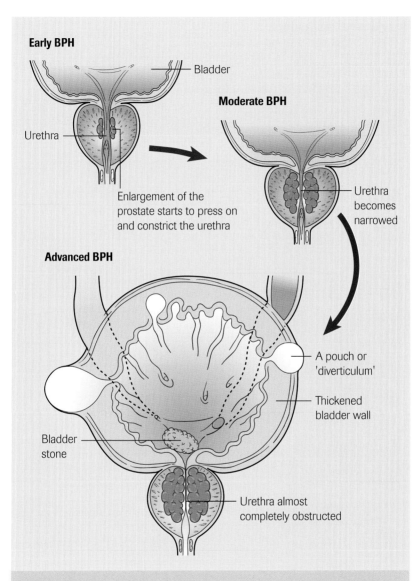

Early BPH

Bladder

Moderate BPH

Urethra

Enlargement of the
prostate starts to press on
and constrict the urethra

Urethra
becomes
narrowed

Advanced BPH

A pouch or
'diverticulum'

Thickened
bladder wall

Bladder
stone

Urethra almost
completely obstructed

BPH arises as a consequence of excess (non-cancerous) growth of prostate tissue. The urethra running through the prostate becomes squeezed and the urine flow becomes obstructed. Because the pressure inside the bladder also builds up, the bladder walls become thickened and diverticula can form. Bladder stones can also occur as a result of this condition

How is BPH diagnosed?

The spectrum of symptoms that are associated with BPH are known collectively as lower urinary tract symptoms (LUTS for short), and are outlined in the table below.

Lower urinary tract symptoms associated with BPH
• Hesitancy (when the urine flow stops and starts)
• A weak urine stream
• You need to strain to pass urine
• Urination takes a long time
• After urinating, you feel like there is still some urine 'left behind' in the bladder
• When you get the urge to urinate, you feel you need to do so urgently
• Frequent trips to the toilet
• Getting up in the night to urinate
• When you get the urge to urinate, you leak a little urine
• A sudden or slowly building inability to urinate

The symptoms of BPH overlap with those of other conditions, so your initial examination should be thorough and your doctor will question you about your general health and symptoms. In order to assess your symptoms systematically, you may be asked questions that relate to a scoring system (an example of this system is shown on page 23). Your doctor will also be concerned with how 'bothersome' you find your symptoms. Again, this can be approached in a systematic manner, and your responses can be scored.

Physical examination and digital rectal examination (DRE)

A DRE will be performed to give the doctor an idea of the size and consistency of your prostate (see pages 21 and 22). He will also feel your abdomen to check whether your bladder is distended so that it can be felt (if it can, this is a sign that you may be retaining urine). Your doctor may also make an assessment of your nervous system, such as testing the muscle tone and sensation in the area around and between the scrotum and anus, as some disorders of the nervous system, such as Parkinson's disease, can give rise to urinary symptoms similar to those of BPH.

Urine test

As a urinary tract infection can cause symptoms such as an increased need to urinate, a urine sample will be checked for signs of bacterial infection or blood.

Blood tests

A very small proportion of men have kidney problems as a consequence of their BPH. By assessing the amount of a substance called creatinine in the blood, your doctor will be able to check whether your kidneys are affected. Your blood sugar level may also be tested to check that you do not have diabetes.

The amount of PSA may also be measured. You might already have read about this in the sections on prostate cancer. PSA is a marker that indicates damage to the prostate, often arising as a result of prostate cancer, but sometimes as a result of BPH. If your PSA level is raised, it may be recommended that you have a prostate biopsy so that prostate cancer can be excluded (see

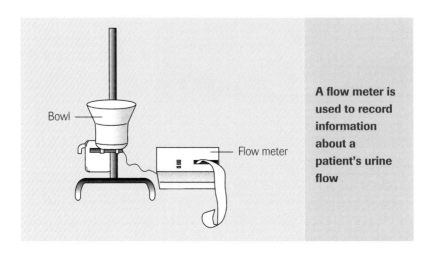

Bowl

Flow meter

A flow meter is used to record information about a patient's urine flow

pages 25 and 26). There is some evidence that your PSA level also gives a rough indication of your prostate size, and this can influence the risk of you developing urinary retention and provide information about the likely success of various treatment options.

Urine flow tests (or uroflowmetry)
By measuring the speed of your urine output over time, your urologist can get some useful information about your urine flow. For this test, you will have to urinate into the bowl of a specialized piece of medical equipment known as a flow meter.

Ultrasound to measure urine left in the bladder
This can give your doctor an idea of how severe the obstruction is and how well you might respond to certain types of treatment. The procedure is very similar to that used with pregnant women. High-frequency sound waves are emitted from a probe that is passed over your abdomen, and the echoes build up a picture that can be seen on a computer monitor.

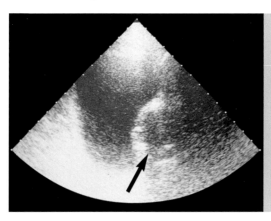

An ultrasound image of the bladder showing that a large volume of urine remains in the bladder after the patient has urinated. In this example, the prostate can be seen bulging into the base of the bladder (arrowed)

Less common tests
Depending on the results from the tests described, your urologist may want to perform some further tests.

Urodynamic measurements are made using a small catheter that is inserted up through the urethra, via your penis, into the bladder. By measuring the pressure within your bladder, your urologist can deduce whether your symptoms are due to BPH or are the result of the bladder itself not working properly. This test is uncomfortable rather than painful, and takes around 20 minutes.

Transrectal ultrasonography (TRUS) is used to visualize the prostate, measure its proportions and to help guide a biopsy needle when there is a possibility of prostate cancer. The procedure is described fully on pages 25 and 26.

Treatment

BPH is usually treated with drugs or surgery. Some men with very mild symptoms opt for watchful waiting, where their condition is monitored so that any worsening of their condition can be quickly spotted and treated. There are also several 'minimally invasive' alternatives, though these are relatively new and long-term experience with them is limited.

Drug treatment

This may be recommended if your symptoms are moderate, though it may also be beneficial for patients with severe symptoms. Certain complications of BPH, such as kidney problems or bladder stones, make surgery a more appropriate option.

There are two main classes of drug that are prescribed for BPH:

- α_1-blockers (referred to as 'alpha-blockers')
- 5α-reductase inhibitors ('five alpha-reductase inhibitors').

α_1-blockers work by helping to relax the muscles at the neck of the bladder and in the prostate (see the diagram overleaf). By reducing the pressure on the urethra, they help to overcome the obstruction and so increase the flow of urine. Results available from studies to date indicate that up to 60% of men find that their symptoms improve significantly within the first 2–3 weeks of treatment with an α_1-blocker.

This type of drug does not cure BPH, but simply helps to alleviate some of the symptoms. You may still develop complications at a later date, and you may still need surgery eventually.

The most commonly occurring side-effects are tiredness, dizziness and headache, which affect around one in ten men. The dosage of earlier α_1-blockers had to be increased gradually to reduce the likelihood of side-effects, but this is not necessary with the more recently developed ones, such as Flomax (tamsulosin) or Xatral (alfuzosin), which seem to have fewer side-effects.

5α-reductase inhibitors work by blocking the conversion of testosterone to another substance, DHT, that is known to have a key role in prostate growth. To date, most information is available on the 5α-reductase inhibitor Proscar; a newer agent, dutasteride, may soon become available. Unlike the α_1-blockers, Proscar does appear to be able to reverse the condition to some extent, particularly if the prostate is significantly enlarged, so its use may reduce the likelihood that you will develop acute urinary retention and eventually require surgery.

The main side-effects of Proscar are a reduced sex drive and difficulty in maintaining/achieving an erection; these appear to

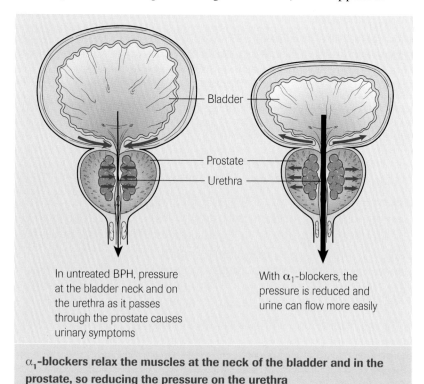

Bladder

Prostate

Urethra

In untreated BPH, pressure at the bladder neck and on the urethra as it passes through the prostate causes urinary symptoms

With α_1-blockers, the pressure is reduced and urine can flow more easily

α_1-blockers relax the muscles at the neck of the bladder and in the prostate, so reducing the pressure on the urethra

affect around 3–5 men in 100. There is a very slight chance that you might experience tenderness around the nipples. These symptoms disappear if treatment is stopped. Be aware that crushed or broken Proscar tablets should not be handled by a woman who is pregnant or who is planning a pregnancy as there is a risk that they could cause problems to a developing baby.

Combination therapy with an α_1-blocker or a 5α-reductase inhibitor has been shown (in the Medical Treatment of Prostate Symptoms study) to be more effective than either agent used alone in preventing the worsening of the symptoms of BPH or the development of complications such as acute retention.

Other medical strategies for symptom relief in BPH include anticholinergic agents like Detrusitol XL (tolterodine) to control urinary urgency and frequency. However, these agents also carry a risk of precipitating acute retention in men with severe obstruction.

In patients who are particularly troubled by the need to pass urine during the night (nocturia), vasopressin analogues such as Desmospray or Desmotabs (desmopressin) last thing at night, used in addition to fluid restriction in the evenings, can be quite effective. These drugs work by reducing the amount of urine produced by the kidneys for 6–8 hours.

Surgery
There are three surgical options for BPH:

- transurethral resection of the prostate (TURP)
- transurethral incision of the prostate (TUIP)
- open prostatectomy.

TURP is the most usual operation, and is usually carried out under a general anaesthetic. It involves passing an instrument that emits a high-frequency current up through the penis, and then using it to cut the middle out of the enlarged prostate, piecemeal (see page 70). A catheter will be passed through the urethra into the bladder at the end of the operation to drain off the urine. This will be left in place for a couple of days. A normal hospital stay following TURP is 3 or 4 days, but you should try to rest as much as possible for a few weeks afterwards to minimize the risks of secondary complications.

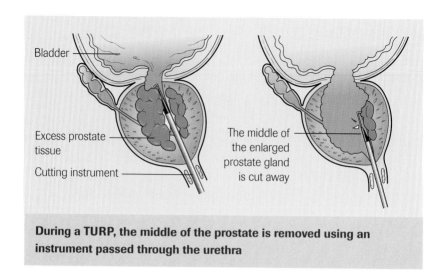

Bladder

Excess prostate tissue

Cutting instrument

The middle of the enlarged prostate gland is cut away

During a TURP, the middle of the prostate is removed using an instrument passed through the urethra

After the operation, you may find that you experience an urgent need to urinate and/or a burning sensation when you pass urine. This should disappear within a few weeks. You may also notice some blood in your urine. This is normal, but if it is particularly heavy or persists for more than a few weeks, or if you notice some blood clots, drink extra fluids and contact your doctor.

The most common side-effect is what is known as retrograde ejaculation – where semen passes into the bladder during orgasm, rather than out through the penis. You then pass the semen mixed with urine next time you urinate. This is not harmful and, providing that they know about this potential side-effect before undergoing the surgery, most men do not find it bothersome. However, retrograde ejaculation may reduce your fertility, but does not make you reliably sterile.

A few men complain of inability to achieve or maintain an erection after the operation, though this does not seem to be a problem specifically caused by this surgical procedure. In a study that compared men with BPH who had undergone a TURP with men with BPH who had not had surgery, the proportions of men who reported erectile problems were similar. Some were even improved by surgery.

A few men notice some incontinence after a TURP – if you find that you are leaking urine slightly, talk to your doctor. This problem nearly always resolves completely with time.

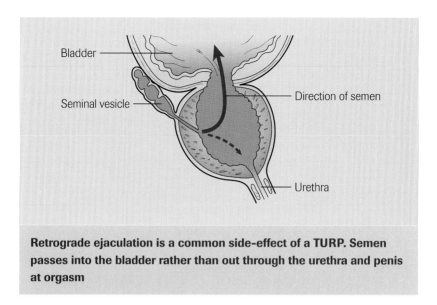

Bladder

Seminal vesicle

Direction of semen

Urethra

Retrograde ejaculation is a common side-effect of a TURP. Semen passes into the bladder rather than out through the urethra and penis at orgasm

An operation under general anaesthetic always carries some small risks, as occasionally an individual reacts badly to being anaesthetized. There is also a small chance of significant blood loss and the subsequent need for a transfusion. These problems are unusual with a TURP, however, and the outcome is usually good.

TUIP is appropriate for the man who is experiencing obstruction problems but who has a relatively small prostate. It is quite quick to perform, taking only around 20 minutes, but you will still be given a general or spinal anaesthetic. As with a TURP, an instrument will be passed up through the penis, but with a TUIP, rather than removing a portion of the prostate, one or two small cuts are made in the neck of the bladder and in the prostate (see page 72). These have the effect of reducing the obstruction and allowing the bladder neck to spring apart. As with a TURP, you will be catheterized at the end of the operation to allow urine to drain away freely. The catheter will be removed after around 24–48 hours, and you will be able to leave hospital after a couple of days. For the next week or so, you should take things easy.

The chance that you will experience a side-effect following a TUIP is lower than following a TURP. Retrograde ejaculation (see page 70), for example, affects a much lower proportion of men after the operation (1 in 10 compared with 7–9 in 10).

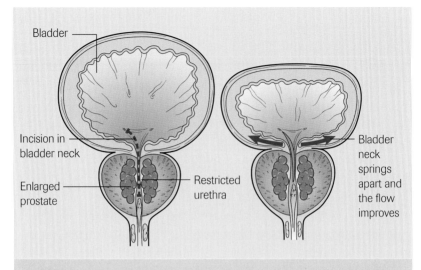

Bladder

Incision in
bladder neck

Enlarged
prostate

Restricted
urethra

Bladder
neck
springs
apart and
the flow
improves

**In TUIP, several small cuts are made in the bladder neck and prostate.
This relieves the pressure on the urethra and urine can flow more
easily**

There is a risk that symptoms will return after the operation
(see table on page 74); if this happens, then it is likely that you
will need a TURP.

Again, as the operation is performed using a general anaesthetic,
there is a small risk of anaesthetic-related complications.

Open prostatectomy is only really appropriate for the man whose
prostate is very large (more than 100 grams) or who has large
bladder stones. It is a more complex procedure than a TURP, and
complications afterwards are somewhat more likely.

The surgeon gains access to the prostate through a horizontal
incision made in the lower abdomen. Through a cut made either in
the prostate or bladder, the surgeon is then able to remove the
central part of the prostate. A catheter will be inserted into your
bladder during the operation so that urine can drain away, and this
will be left in place for 3 or 4 days. Because this is relatively major
surgery, you will usually need to stay in hospital for about a week.
Even when you go home, you are advised to rest for up to 6 weeks,
and you should avoid doing heavy lifting for several months. The
operation will leave a scar.

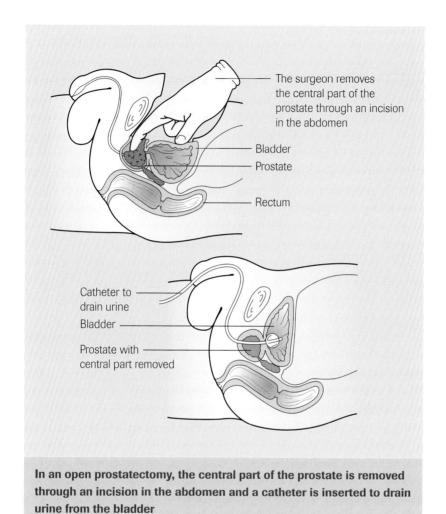

The surgeon removes the central part of the prostate through an incision in the abdomen

Bladder

Prostate

Rectum

Catheter to drain urine

Bladder

Prostate with central part removed

In an open prostatectomy, the central part of the prostate is removed through an incision in the abdomen and a catheter is inserted to drain urine from the bladder

An open prostatectomy can also result in retrograde ejaculation (see page 70), with about 7 in 10 men being affected; some men also find it difficult to achieve/maintain an erection (around 2 men in 10). The risks associated with surgery of this type are discussed in the TURP section.

The long-term picture following surgery

Useful information comparing the outcomes following each surgical procedure is presented in the table overleaf.

Outcome after the three main surgical options for treatment of BPH			
	TURP	TUIP	Open prostatectomy
Likelihood that symptoms will improve	90%	80%	98%
Usual reduction in symptom score (see page 23)	85%	73%	79%
Likelihood that you will need further surgery within 8 years	16–20%	Over 20%	10%

Watchful waiting

This may be recommended if your symptoms are mild or if you are not too troubled by them. Your doctor will advise you about small changes that you can make to your lifestyle that might help; for example, try not to drink large volumes of fluid in the evenings. Tea, coffee and alcohol can worsen symptoms. At regular intervals (usually yearly), you will have a check up that will include the examination and tests described on pages 20–22.

Minimally invasive treatments

As has already been said, these are relatively new. While greeted with enthusiasm by some urologists – and many patients – it has to be said that currently minimally invasive techniques do not seem to work as well (or as definitively) as the more traditional treatments. Two that deserve a mention are transurethral microwave thermotherapy and laser therapy.

Transurethral microwave thermotherapy involves using microwave energy to generate heat, which then destroys some of the prostate tissue. Under local anaesthetic, the microwave device is inserted up through the urethra inside a catheter; the temperature of surrounding tissues is monitored using a probe inserted in the rectum.

Laser therapy is carried out under general anaesthetic. A laser probe is inserted up through the penis, and the laser energy it generates destroys some of the prostate tissue. Catheterization is necessary for a few days afterwards. A new holmium laser technique allows pieces of prostate to be cut away, and these pieces are then removed from the bladder, rather as happens during a TURP. Bleeding is less common with laser therapy, but a burning sensation on passing urine may be prolonged and quite troublesome.

Plant extracts (phytotherapy)

There is an increasing range of plant extracts available that supposedly alleviate BPH, and many claims have been made for their effectiveness. However, scientific data from properly conducted, long-term studies to support their usefulness are limited, and many doctors believe that the extracts just have a placebo effect, although some patients swear by them. Nevertheless, they almost certainly do no harm.

Prevention

Although we have still to identify the fundamental steps in the development of BPH, we know that testosterone is certainly involved in some way (and it is likely that the female hormone oestrogen also has a role). Epidemiological data suggest that men in the Far East are protected, to some extent, against the risks of BPH by minute amounts of oestrogen-like substances in the food that they eat (for example, soya contains the phytoestrogen genistein). This raises the question as to whether dietary supplements taken regularly by men in Europe, the USA and elsewhere could protect against the risk of this disease. Long-term studies involving many men are needed to confirm this.

Frequently asked questions about BPH

What causes BPH? It's caused by a non-cancerous overgrowth of tissue in the middle part of the prostate, but we don't know what actually starts this process off or allows it to progress. We do know that the male hormone testosterone is involved, as men who have been castrated at an early age (and so don't produce testosterone) never develop BPH. We also know that testosterone triggers the release of substances in the body called growth factors which can stimulate tissue growth. But why this happens in some men but not others is still not clear. The condition does seem to run in families.

Which are the worst symptoms? Many men find that having to get up and go to the toilet at night is the most troublesome aspect of this condition, as it makes them tired during the day. Having to urinate frequently during the day, sometimes with a sense of urgency, can also be trying for patients, and can make travelling or attending events, such as the theatre or cinema, rather difficult.

Can I ignore my symptoms? If you've read this far, you'll know that the symptoms of BPH can be similar to those of prostate cancer. For this reason alone you should see your GP. Even if you do have BPH, an enlarged prostate can cause knock-on effects in the bladder and kidneys. Pouches called 'diverticula' can form in the bladder and can predispose you to urinary infections (cystitis). Bladder stones can also form, and can be painful, while continued obstruction of the urethra can cause kidney damage, which may be permanent. The moral of the story is see your doctor sooner rather than later!

What should I do if I am suddenly unable to pass urine? Acute urinary retention (the sudden, painful inability to urinate) is a common complication of BPH. It is usually, but not always, preceded by symptoms of prostatic obstruction. If you find that you cannot pass urine at all, contact your doctor or go to your nearest

Accident & Emergency Department. Try to drink less fluid because your bladder will already be uncomfortably full. Tell the doctor and nurses how much discomfort you are in so that you do not wait longer than necessary to have a catheter passed via the penis to drain your overdistended bladder. After this, you will usually be admitted to hospital. Often the doctor will remove the catheter after an α-blocker has been given orally to see if you can pass urine normally. If retention recurs, another catheter will be put in and then you will either be scheduled to have a TURP within the next few days, or sent home with a catheter in place, to await readmission for an operation to restore normal voiding.

So what should I look out for? Regularly having to get up more than once a night to urinate can be a sign that your bladder is not emptying properly. You may notice that your urine stream isn't what it used to be in terms of volume or 'force', and/or you may develop a urinary infection (which will make you want to urinate often, give you a burning sensation when you urinate, and possibly also a temperature). Finally, if you pass blood in your urine, see your doctor urgently.

Why would I be referred to a specialist? BPH can often be managed by your GP, but some men will be referred to a specialist urologist. You'll usually be referred if:

- your symptoms appeared suddenly or are severe
- you have had repeated urinary infections
- you have passed blood in your urine
- your PSA level is over 4 ng/mL
- your GP thinks you may have a bladder stone
- the results from your blood tests suggest you might have kidney damage.

What will the specialist do? He'll ask about your symptoms and examine you. To see how efficiently you are emptying your bladder you will probably have a flow test and ultrasound. Your PSA level may be rechecked, and if it's found to be higher than normal (that is, above 4 ng/mL), you may have a transrectal ultrasound-guided biopsy to check that the swelling is not cancerous.

77

These tests are not unduly uncomfortable. Nobody enjoys a digital rectal examination, but it's over in a few seconds. The flow test and bladder ultrasound are totally painless. Only a proportion of patients need a biopsy, and the procedure is now much less uncomfortable with the use of local anaesthetic – it is certainly worth asking for this.

Which drug is best for BPH? α_1-blockers such as Flomax, Xatral and Cardura (doxazosin) all act quickly to relieve symptoms regardless of the size of your prostate. 5α-reductase inhibitors such as Proscar (finasteride) work more slowly, but as they seem to shrink the prostate, they seem to help avoid complications and reduce the need for surgery. α_1-blockers therefore are a 'quick fix' but do not cure the underlying problem. 5α-reductase inhibitors work better in patients with larger glands, but take 6 months or so to become effective.

Are microwave and laser treatments safe? And do they work? A great deal of work has gone into developing alternatives to traditional surgery. Both microwave and laser treatment appear to be safe and they probably have less effect on ejaculation than TURP. In terms of how well they work, results with these techniques are improving as the technology develops, but heat-based treatments such as these still do not produce the rapid and reliable results achieved with TURP.

What can go wrong if I opt for a TURP? Although this procedure is largely safe and effective, complications can occasionally occur (as with any operation). The main problem is bleeding, either at the time of the surgery or afterwards. It can usually be dealt with by washing out the area with relatively large volumes of liquid (irrigation and bladder washouts), but sometimes the patient needs a second anaesthetic and a telescopic examination (cystoscopy) to find and repair by diathermy the source of the bleeding. In the longer term, incontinence after a TURP is quite rare but does affect a tiny proportion of men, as does scarring (stricture) of the urethra, which may need further surgery to remedy.

How will having a TURP affect my sex life? It shouldn't affect your sex drive, erection or sensation at orgasm, but it will mean that you have a dry orgasm with no ejaculate. This doesn't usually bother patients as long as they know about it before they have the surgery. If it was OK before the operation, most men report that their sex life after a TURP is quite satisfactory. In addition, you should need to get up less often during the night to urinate, and should have an improved urinary stream.

What are the chances that I'll need a second operation? Because the prostate continues to grow after a TURP, a proportion of men will need a second operation eventually. One man in ten undergoing TURP will need a second operation sometime during the following 5 years.

What questions should I put to my urologist before I agree to surgery? Ask him who will actually carry out the operation, how many times that person has performed the same type of surgery, and what his results are. You are looking for an experienced surgeon (one who has carried out the operation at least 100 times previously) who has a high rate of success and a low rate of complications. Also ask how long you'll have to wait for your operation, and check the cancellation rate (through bed shortages). If you find it difficult to ask the surgeon these questions directly, you can always telephone his secretary and ask her.

What should I discuss at my follow-up visit? The most important thing to check is the results from the pathology laboratory, where they will have examined, under a microscope, the pieces of prostate tissue removed during the TURP. Most men (nine out of ten) undergoing TURP will simply have signs of BPH. But one man in ten also has small quantities of prostate cancer in the tissue fragments. If this is the case, further investigations will be needed, such as a PSA check and, possibly, further biopsies from the remaining prostate tissue; depending on these results, further treatment may be necessary.

After prostate surgery your flow rate should be much stronger, but frequency and urgency of urination take longer to improve. Tell your doctor about your symptoms and ask him how long it will be before everything is back to normal.

The painful prostate: prostatitis

Prostatitis literally means 'inflammation of the prostate'. In fact, by no means every patient suffering from prostatitis actually has an inflamed prostate, so the name is slightly misleading. In the UK, the condition accounts for almost one-quarter of all consultations with a urologist.

Patients with prostatitis often suffer pain and discomfort in the area around and between the anus and scrotum, and just above the pubic bone. Men with the condition may have to urinate frequently and this can be very inconvenient. There may also be a burning sensation at the time of urination and/or some discomfort during or after ejaculation (see the table below for a more complete list of symptoms). Although prostatitis is often considered to be the result of a bacterial infection in the prostate, inflammation, when present, more commonly occurs spontaneously. Some studies suggest that in the absence of infection, inflammation may result from urine

Symptoms of prostatitis

- Chills and fever

- Pain in:
  - lower back (may be particularly painful after sex)
  - between the scrotum and rectum
  - penis
  - prostate (felt as lower abdominal pain and pain in the area between the scrotum and anus)
  - testicles
  - rectum
  - inner thighs

- Pain/difficulty in passing urine

- A need for frequent urination

being forced backwards up the prostatic ducts at the time of urination.

Even when infection is the source of inflammation, it may be difficult to eradicate because the bacteria responsible tend to be inaccessible to antibiotics. This is because they usually lurk deep inside the prostate (for example, the bacteria may be inside the tiny stones that form in the prostatic ducts).

Risk factors

Men who have an increased risk of prostatitis include those who have long-term catheterization and those who have urinary tract infections that remain untreated. Unprotected anal intercourse is another risk factor for this condition. Prostatitis most commonly affects men in the age range 30–50 years, but a man of any age can be affected. Most affected men have no identifiable risk factors.

Tests

Because prostatitis is often the result of a bacterial infection, your doctor will usually want to check a sample of your urine and prostatic secretions for bacteria (the sample will be sent to the laboratory for analysis, so you will not get the results straight away).

Obtaining a sample of prostatic secretions

You'll be asked to pass urine and provide a sample, and then your prostate will be massaged (see page 82) so that secretions are released. These will be collected from the urethra into a sterile pot. Finally, a second urine sample will be collected. If there is a bacterial infection, bacteria can be grown up in the laboratory from cultures of the prostatic secretions and the second urine sample. This method also allows the specific type of bacteria responsible to be identified, and an appropriate antibiotic to be prescribed.

Other tests

Depending on your symptoms, your doctor may also check that you don't have BPH or prostate cancer – the tests that may be performed are discussed on pages 20–22 and 64–67. Remember that prostatitis, particularly when the inflammation is severe, may sometimes cause a temporary increase in blood PSA level (see page 14). Prostatitis can also cause blood flow in the prostate to become increased, and this can show up when a transrectal ultrasound study of the prostate is performed using what is known as a colour Doppler probe.

Treatment

If a bacterial infection is the cause of your symptoms, you will be prescribed a course of antibiotics. You may need to take these for a relatively long period, often 4–6 weeks, and it is very important that you complete the course (the diagram opposite explains why this is so). You may also be prescribed an anti-inflammatory drug, such as Voltarol (diclofenac), to reduce the inflammation in the prostate.

If bacteria are not present, you may be given an anti-inflammatory drug. You may also find that prostatic massage performed by your doctor helps (see the diagram below).

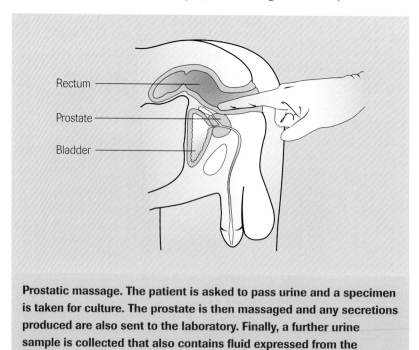

Rectum

Prostate

Bladder

Prostatic massage. The patient is asked to pass urine and a specimen is taken for culture. The prostate is then massaged and any secretions produced are also sent to the laboratory. Finally, a further urine sample is collected that also contains fluid expressed from the prostate

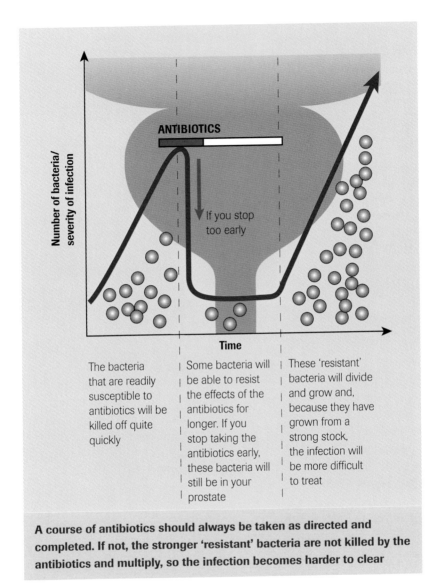

Number of bacteria/ severity of infection

ANTIBIOTICS

If you stop too early

Time

| The bacteria that are readily susceptible to antibiotics will be killed off quite quickly | Some bacteria will be able to resist the effects of the antibiotics for longer. If you stop taking the antibiotics early, these bacteria will still be in your prostate | These 'resistant' bacteria will divide and grow and, because they have grown from a strong stock, the infection will be more difficult to treat |

A course of antibiotics should always be taken as directed and completed. If not, the stronger 'resistant' bacteria are not killed by the antibiotics and multiply, so the infection becomes harder to clear

Antibiotics can also be helpful in these circumstances, perhaps because the cultures do not tell the whole story.

Prostatitis, though troublesome, is not a life-threatening condition and is not a precursor to BPH or prostate cancer. You may find that, over the years, the prostatitis returns from time to time (particularly if the condition has a non-bacterial cause), but your doctor should be able to help alleviate the symptoms quite effectively, so don't suffer in silence.

Prostatic abscess

Occasionally prostatitis with a bacterial cause can lead to the formation of an abscess within the prostate itself. If this is the case, your doctor may need to take a sample of fluid from the abscess and will do so using ultrasound for guidance (see page 25). The sample can then be checked to see what type of bacteria has caused the infection, so that appropriate antibiotics can be given.

Abscesses sometimes have to be drained, which involves passing an instrument up through the penis under anaesthetic, making a small cut through to the abscess and then 'nicking' the abscess to allow pus to drain out. A course of antibiotics and a period of catheterization are also usually necessary.

Preventing prostatitis

Prostatitis is the affliction of the prostate about which we know least. So, not surprisingly, we currently have little idea how to prevent the problem. The best advice at present is to avoid the risk factors for prostatitis where possible (for example, if you have symptoms of a urinary tract infection, such as a burning sensation when urinating, or cloudy, smelly urine, visit your doctor and complete any prescribed courses of antibiotics). Also, maintain a healthy lifestyle, eat a diet low in saturated fats, take plenty of exercise and wear a condom if you have anal sex.

Pain but no inflammation: prostatodynia

Some men feel pain that appears to come from their prostate or the surrounding area but on investigation, there doesn't appear to be any inflammation or infection. What causes this condition, which is referred to as prostatodynia or pelvic pain syndrome, is not known, though it may result from spasm of the pelvic muscles brought on by stress or anxiety. Depending on your symptoms, you may be given α_1-blockers (see page 67), which will have to be taken for some time. More research is needed into this disorder to improve the quality of life of those affected.

Frequently asked questions about prostatitis

Why does it tend to affect younger men? No one knows why some men get prostatitis and others do not. The prostate is certainly more prone to inflammation than almost any other part of the body, and one theory is that urine may track backwards into the prostate during urination, causing an inflammatory response. We still don't know why younger men seem to be more prone to the disease or why it recurs so often.

My doctor has referred to different categories of prostatitis. What are they and which one have I got? An American body, the National Institutes of Health, has recently produced the following classification of prostatitis:

- Category I: acute bacterial prostatitis
- Category II: chronic bacterial prostatitis
- Category III: chronic prostatitis/chronic pelvic pain syndrome
  - IIIA: inflammatory
  - IIIB: non-inflammatory
- Category IV: asymptomatic inflammatory prostatitis.

As to which category you belong to, the important considerations are whether the problem is acute (comes on quickly) or chronic and relapsing (where you have the symptoms for a long time or have regular bouts), and whether it is caused by a specific infection. In order to answer this second question, a sample of prostatic secretions obtained by massaging the prostate will be sent to the laboratory for analysis (the lower tract localization test or LTLT).

How uncomfortable are the tests for prostatitis? Testing for prostatitis often involves a prostatic massage. This is unquestionably uncomfortable, but not actually painful. You'll also probably have transrectal ultrasound, which has a similar level of discomfort. Occasionally, a test known as 'urodynamics' is needed, which involves passing a small catheter into the bladder via the penis and the insertion into the rectum of a small tube to monitor pressure. The bladder is then filled with a fluid that will show up on X-ray, and you'll be asked to pass urine. While you're doing this, the pressure in the bladder is recorded and the process can be visualized on an X-ray screen. In this way, your doctor can check whether there is anything obstructing the urine flow.

What treatment is right for me and are there any side-effects? If there is a bacterial cause of your prostatitis, you'll be given a prolonged course of antibiotics. Even when there are no signs of bacteria, some men still respond favourably to antibiotics. You'll also probably be prescribed an anti-inflammatory drug to try to reduce the inflammation.

Ciproxin (ciprofloxacin) is an antibiotic commonly prescribed for prostatitis, and if you are taking this, avoid sunbathing, as it can increase the sensitivity of your skin. Most anti-inflammatory drugs can cause indigestion or even peptic ulcers and bleeding in the stomach, and the tablets should be taken with meals to help avoid this. Report any stomach pains to your doctor and stop taking the tablets immediately.

If the symptoms resolve with treatment, what are the chances of them returning? Unfortunately, quite high, as prostatitis has a pronounced tendency to recur. If you do suffer further attacks, see your doctor straight away as prompt treatment can help to stop the infection or inflammation from taking hold.

Can I help myself to avoid the chances of a repeat attack? The usual health advice is appropriate here – lots of exercise and a healthy diet. A healthy immune system should help you fight off infections. Some doctors advise their patients with a history of prostatitis to take vitamins D and E, selenium and zinc supplements, but there is little firm evidence to support their usefulness in avoiding prostatitis.

Is prostatitis sexually transmitted? In some cases it is, theoretically at least. In practice, however, prostatitis seldom results from sexual activity, so there is little logic in treating your partner (though very occasionally this may be recommended depending on the bacterial cause).

Does having chronic prostatitis make me more likely to have other prostate problems? In theory, long-term inflammation could promote the development of cancer, but there is no evidence to suggest that this actually happens. Similarly, there is nothing to suggest that BPH is more common among prostatitis sufferers. Fortunately, the condition tends to burn itself out and resolve over time.

Appendix: some practical advice

Prostate Research Campaign UK thanks Jane Dawoodi, a Nurse Specialist, for contributing this section.

Emergency? When to call your doctor

- If you have BPH, and find that you suddenly cannot pass urine (you will be in a fair amount of pain).
- If you have had a biopsy or operation, and develop symptoms of infection:
  - high temperature
  - pain on urination
  - cloudy, smelly urine
  - swollen or painful testicles.
- If you have a catheter in place and notice that urine does not drain into the collecting bag for 4 hours or more.
- If you suddenly start to pass blood in your urine. Drink extra fluids and call your doctor. If clots start to form, there is a risk that you will be unable to pass urine, in which case you will need to go to hospital urgently to have a catheter inserted via the penis to drain urine from your bladder.

Having an operation
Consent

By signing a consent form, you are formally agreeing to undergo the treatment specified on the form. So do not sign it lightly.

- Be sure that you know what the operation involves, what the side-effects and risks are, and what effect the operation will have on the course of your illness.
- Be aware that you may need to undergo an investigation of your prostate and bladder carried out under general anaesthetic.
- Ask who will be performing the surgery.

If you are not completely satisfied, do not sign the form.

Talking to the anaesthetist

Before your operation, you will meet your anaesthetist. He is a fully trained doctor who has specialized in the administration of anaesthetics. You might be asked some of the following questions about your medical history.

- Have you had surgery before? If so, were there any problems or complications?
- Has any member of your family had a problem following an operation?
- Are you taking any medicines that have been prescribed to you or that you bought from a chemist, such as aspirin?
- Do you or any member of your family have any allergies (for example, to plasters or antibiotics)?
- Do you have any back, chest or heart problems?
- Do you smoke?

The anaesthetist will also ask about your teeth. This may seem a strange line of questioning, but he needs to know whether there is anything in your mouth, such as a cap or a crown, that might come loose during the operation.

Don't be afraid to ask him about any questions or concerns that you may have.

Looking after a catheter

If you have a catheter inserted during surgery (for example following a radical prostatectomy), and have to keep it for a few days after you have been sent home, it is important to keep it clean. The hospital staff will probably have shown you how to do this, so this short section should act as a reminder.

The catheter itself

This just needs to be kept clean. Always wash your hands before touching it or any part of the system. Twice a day, wash the area of skin where the catheter enters your body with soap and water, and then dry it thoroughly. Don't use anything else, such as talc, around this area.

The catheter is held in place by a Velcro strap, which fits around the catheter and your leg, and prevents it from being pulled.

The leg bag

This is securely attached to your leg by a leg-bag support, which is rather like a sock. The leg bag will fill with urine during the day and you will feel it getting heavier as it fills. Don't let it become too full – open the tap over the toilet and drain the urine from the bag at regular intervals. Always wash your hands before and after doing this.

The night bag

This should be attached to the bottom of the leg bag, and the tap should be opened to allow urine to drain into the night bag, which should be attached to a stand (you will have to be shown how to do this). In the morning, don't forget to close the tap before removing the night bag. After disposing of the urine, rinse the night bag with warm water so that it is ready to be used again the next night.

Changing bags

Unless there is a problem, only change your catheter bag once a week. To dispose of a bag, empty it, rinse it out and put it in a sealed plastic bag with your household waste.

Leakage

This can occur as a result of an abdominal cramp (actually a bladder spasm). If you leak a little urine outside of the catheter, check that the connection between the catheter and the leg bag is still good and that urine is still being collected in the leg bag. If it is, then carry on as normal, but let your doctor or nurse know what has happened.

If urine is not collecting in the bag

Check that:

- the bag is below the level of your bladder (if, for example, you are using the night bag on the stand)
- there are no twists or kinks in the catheter.

Also ask yourself whether you have been drinking sufficient fluids or whether you are constipated, as this can be a sign that you are dehydrated.

If 1–2 hours pass without any urine draining into the bag, contact your doctor or nurse immediately – the catheter may have become blocked, in which case it will have to be flushed or changed.

Blood in the urine

This is common after radical prostatectomy. As you become more mobile, the catheter can irritate the bladder and lead to blood in the urine. You may also see blood in the urine when you open your bowels. Don't worry about it unless you can see large clots or pieces of tissue passing down the catheter. These can cause a blockage and you should contact your doctor or nurse for advice.

Infections

You should contact your doctor if you have any of the following symptoms, as they may be due to infection:

- cloudy urine
- a burning sensation (cystitis)
- strong-smelling urine
- a high temperature.

Eating and drinking

If you have had an operation, you will probably feel sore. It's therefore a good idea to eat foods that will help you to avoid constipation, so that you don't have to strain to empty your bowels. Eat sensibly, including plenty of fresh and dried fruit (for example, prunes), fresh vegetables, wholemeal bread and high-fibre breakfast cereals, such as All-Bran, in your diet.

Also keep your fluid intake up – try to drink 2 litres (3½ pints) a day if possible. This may take a bit of readjustment as you might have reduced the amount you drank before your operation in an effort to keep the number of trips to the toilet down. Water or flavoured squash drinks are fine, but try not to overdo your intake of tea, coffee or cola. It's also worth trying cranberry juice, as this probably reduces the likelihood of urinary tract infections (it is thought to work by making the environment of the bladder and urethra unfavourable to bacteria).

Advice about continence

Incontinence pads

You'll probably need to wear a small incontinence pad for a few weeks after a radical prostatectomy. These will be supplied by the hospital, and further supplies are available from your GP or can be bought from chemists.

Pelvic floor exercises

If you have had a radical prostatectomy, pelvic floor exercises will help you to regain your continence control. First you need to become aware of your pelvic floor muscles. Do this in two stages. While passing urine, contract the muscles up and inwards to stop the flow. Then let go. It doesn't matter if the flow does not stop altogether. The important thing is recognizing the muscles you are using. Once you have done this, there is no need to keep stopping and starting the urine flow. Secondly, tighten the rest of your pelvic floor muscles by pulling up the muscles around your rectum as if to control an attack of diarrhoea.

You should use all of these muscles at the same time when performing pelvic floor exercise. Draw them up and hold them for a count of five, and repeat until you have done five contractions. Do 20 short, sharp contractions daily. Try to keep your stomach, thigh and buttock muscles relaxed so that you use only your pelvic floor muscles.

Do these exercises once each hour every day. You will probably need to do the regular exercises for several weeks before you notice any improvement. To help you remember to do your exercises, try to schedule each set of contractions to accompany a certain daily task to build them into your routine.

After starting the exercise programme, you may notice a mild aching sensation as the muscles get tired. The ache should disappear within a few days, but you can take a rest from the exercises for a day or two if you wish. However, if you are at all concerned, you should consult your doctor.

Coping with impotence

Some treatments for prostate cancer and BPH can leave you with impotence (or erectile dysfunction), although orgasm is usually unaffected. Several options to help overcome this problem are now available, with the best known being Viagra® (sildenafil). Clive Turner, in his section answering commonly asked questions, looks at this subject in more detail (see pages 59–60). Talk to your doctor if you experience impotence after treatment. He will be able to advise you about the appropriate options, and give you further information about the pros and cons. As Clive Turner stresses in his section, don't buy Viagra on the 'black market' – always go through your doctor. If Viagra does not help, there are other options, such as Uprima or prostaglandin injections, which your doctor will be able to discuss with you.

Appendix: commonly used medication

α_1-blockers are used in BPH to help to relax the muscles in the bladder and the prostate, which in turn helps to reduce the pressure on the urethra.

5α-reductase inhibitors are used in BPH to block the conversion of testosterone to another substance, DHT, which appears to stimulate overgrowth of prostate tissue.

LHRH analogues are used in prostate cancer to 'switch off' testosterone production.

Anti-androgens are used in prostate cancer to block the action of testosterone.

Anticholinergics and antispasmodics are used in BPH to treat irritative symptoms including urinary frequency and urgency.

Vasopressin analogues are used in BPH to reduce the amount of urine produced at night, thus reducing the need to get out of bed to pass urine.

	Brand names	Recommended doses
α_1-blockers		
Indoramin	Doralese	20 mg twice daily
Prazosin	Hypovase	500 µg twice daily
Doxazosin	Cardura XL	4–8 mg/day
Alfuzosin	Xatral XL	10 mg/day
Terazosin	Hytrin	2–10 mg/day
Tamsulosin	Flomax MR	400 µg/day

	Brand names	Recommended doses
5α-reductase inhibitors		
Finasteride	Proscar	5 mg/day
LHRH analogues		
Goserelin	Zoladex	3.6 mg/month or 10.8 mg 3 monthly
Buserelin	Suprefact	500 µg three times daily for 7 days
Leuprorelin	Prostap SR	3.75 mg/month or 11.25 mg 3 monthly
Triptorelin	Decapeptyl SR	3 mg every 4 weeks
Anti-androgens		
Cyproterone acetate	Cyprostat	100 mg three times daily
Flutamide	Chimax	250 mg three times daily
	Drogenil	250 mg three times daily
Bicalutamide	Casodex	50–150 mg/day
Anticholinergics and antispasmodics		
Flaxovate	Urispas	200 µg three times daily
Oxybutynin	Cystrin	3 mg twice daily
	Ditropan XL	2.5 mg twice daily
Propiverine	Detrunorm	15 mg twice daily
Tolterodine	Detrusitol XL	4 mg/day
Trospium	Regurin	20 mg twice daily
Vasopressin analogues		
Desmopressin	DDVAP nasal	10–20 µg at bedtime
	Desmospray	10–20 µg at bedtime
	Desmotabs	200 µg at bedtime
Anti-inflammatory agents		
For example:		
Diclofenac	Voltarol SR	75 mg/day
Antibiotics		
For example:		
Ciprofloxacin	Ciproxin	500 mg twice daily

Appendix: useful resources

Charities and support groups

Prostate Research Campaign UK
PO Box 2371
Swindon SN1 3WJ
Email: info@prostate-research.org.uk
www.prostate-research.org.uk

CancerBACUP
3 Bath Place
Rivington Street
London EC2A 3JR
Information service: 020 7613 2121
Free helpline 0808 800 1234
www.bacup.org.uk

Cancerlink
11–21 Northdown Street
London N1 9BN
Free helpline: 0808 808 0000

The Impotence Association
PO Box 10296
London SW17 9WH
Helpline: 020 8767 7791
www.impotence.org.uk

The Continence Foundation
307 Hatton Square
16 Baldwins Gardens
London EC1N 7RJ
Helpline: 020 7831 9831 (9.30 am – 4.30 pm, Monday to Friday)
www.continence-foundation.org.uk

The Men's Health Forum
Tavistock House
Tavistock Square
London WC1H 9HR
www.menshealthforum.org.uk

Internet sites

There is a wealth of information on the internet, but tread carefully – sites are unregulated. Look for information that is supported by scientific studies or presented by reputable sources.

Some useful UK sites are:

- Prostate Research Campaign UK at www.prostate-research.org.uk

- Cancer BACUP at www.bacup.org.uk

- The Impotence Association at www.impotence.org.uk

- The Continence Foundation at www.continence-foundation.org.uk

- Patient UK at www.patient.org.uk

- Embarrassing Problems at www.embarrassingproblems.com

Guide to medical terms

α_1**-blockers:** one of the two types of drug usually prescribed for BPH. They work by helping to relax muscles in the bladder and prostate, which in turn helps to reduce the pressure on the urethra.

5α-reductase inhibitors: one of the two types of drug usually prescribed for BPH. They work by blocking the conversion of testosterone to another substance, DHT, which appears to stimulate overgrowth of prostate tissue.

Advanced: cancer is described as advanced when it has spread beyond the site where it started. Prostate cancer is described as being **locally advanced** when it has invaded parts of the body around the prostate. When the cancer has begun to spread to more distant sites, such as the bones, it is no longer localized and so is referred to as **advanced**.

Alpha-blockers: *see* α_1-blockers.

Angiogenesis: the development of a blood supply. As a tumour grows, the formation of a blood supply is vital to cancer cells so that they can survive and divide. Researchers are currently developing drugs that could hinder angiogenesis, and so stop cancers growing.

Anti-androgens: drugs that may be prescribed to combat prostate cancer. They work by blocking the action of testosterone, which appears to stimulate the growth of prostate cancer.

Anticholinergic agents: drugs sometimes used to control urinary urgency and frequency associated with BPH.

Benign: non-cancerous. An area of unregulated tissue growth that does not have the capacity to invade surrounding healthy tissue or metastasize.

Biopsy: a sample of tissue taken from the body. Biopsies of prostate tissue are checked in the laboratory for signs of cancer.

Bone scan: a means of seeing whether the cancer has spread to the bones. It involves injecting the patient with a radioactive material that then spreads around the body. The final pattern of distribution will highlight any areas where cancer may be developing.

BPH (benign prostatic hyperplasia): a non-cancerous condition that causes the prostate to become enlarged, which may lead to difficulty with urination.

Brachytherapy: a type of radiotherapy for prostate cancer in which radioactive pellets are implanted into the prostate.

Cancerous: refers to unregulated tissue growth that has developed the ability to invade surrounding healthy tissue.

Catheter: a narrow tube inserted into the penis and up into the bladder to drain urine away. A catheter may be inserted during an operation so that the bladder doesn't fill with urine while the surgeon is working on it. It may be left in place for some time afterwards so that the patient can pass urine while his urethra and bladder heal. Sometimes catheters are also inserted via the penis so that fluid can be passed into the bladder; for example, see urodynamics.

Cavernous nerves: the nerves involved in sexual arousal and erection that lie close to the prostate. They may be disturbed during radical prostatectomy.

Cells: tiny, specialized units from which the body is built. Healthy cells grow and divide as part of their normal lifecycle; in cancer, these processes get out of control because the usual mechanisms that keep them in check have broken down.

Chemotherapy: the use of drugs to destroy cancer cells.

Continence: the ability to maintain control over bladder and bowel emptying.

CT scanning: a method of using sequential X-rays to build up a three-dimensional picture of the body. CT stands for 'computed tomography'.

Cystoscopy: the use of a telescope to examine the inside of the bladder.

DHT: the male hormone testosterone can be converted in the body to DHT, which is thought to stimulate the growth of prostate tissue. DHT stands for 'dihydrotestosterone'.

Differentiated (as in 'well, moderately well or poorly differentiated'): a term used to describe healthy, organized tissue. As cancer invades, the tissue structure becomes disorganized or **de-differentiated**, and looks less and less like normal tissue.

DRE (digital rectal examination): a procedure that allows the doctor to assess the size and texture of the patient's prostate gland. It involves placing a finger into the patient's back passage (rectum) and feeling (palpating) the gland.

Gland: a group of cells with the specialized function of making a particular fluid or secretion. The fluid made in the prostate mixes with the jelly-like storage form of the sperm to make semen, which can then be ejaculated.

Gleason score: a number from 2 to 10 that is used as an indicator of how aggressive the patient's cancer is. The score is derived from an assessment (Gleason grade) of two areas of a sample (biopsy) of prostate tissue (e.g. 3 + 4 = 7).

Grade: how the prostate tissue appears under a microscope. The more aggressive the cancer, the less it looks like normal prostate tissue. The Gleason grading system uses a scale of 1–5, with 5 indicating the most aggressive-looking cancer.

Hormones: usually described as 'chemical messengers', these substances can influence processes at different sites in the body. Testosterone is a well-known hormone that influences many aspects of 'maleness'.

Hormone therapy: the use of drugs to block the stimulatory effects of testosterone on the growth of prostate tissue. Technically, orchidectomy can also be described as hormone therapy, as the testicles are removed so that testosterone is no longer produced.

Impotence (or erectile dysfunction): a state in which an erection cannot be achieved and/or maintained.

LHRH analogues: drugs used in hormone therapy for prostate cancer. They work by switching off testosterone production. LHRH stands for 'luteinizing hormone releasing hormone'.

LUTS: lower urinary tract symptoms. The term used to describe the range of symptoms associated with BPH.

Lymph nodes: these occur at intervals throughout the lymphatic system and act as filters, so cells such as cancer cells tend to accumulate at these points. A well-known example of the lymph nodes (or 'glands') lie in the neck just below the jaw; these tend to become swollen during flu-type illnesses.

Lymphatic system: a network of vessels that drain fluid (lymph) from the body's organs so that it can be filtered and returned to the blood.

Malignant: *see* cancerous.

Maximal androgen blockade: the use of LHRH analogues and long-term anti-androgens to help slow the progression of prostate cancer.

Metastases: secondary cancers that occur at sites distant from the original cancer. The cancer has the ability to **metastasize** when cells can break off from the primary tumour and establish secondary tumours at other sites.

MRI: a means of building up a three-dimensional picture of the body using magnetic fields. MRI stands for 'magnetic resonance imaging'.

Oncologist: a doctor who specializes in the medical treatment of cancer.

Open prostatectomy: an operation for BPH that involves removing the central part of the prostate. Access is gained via an incision through the abdominal wall.

Orchidectomy: an operation for prostate cancer in which both testicles are removed from the scrotum so that testosterone production ceases.

Palliative care: this becomes important in the later stages of cancer where the aim of the medical team is to make the patient as comfortable as possible.

Pathologist: a doctor who examines tissue samples microscopically to obtain information to help with diagnosis and treatment.

Pelvic pain syndrome: *see* prostatodynia.

Perineum: the area around and between the scrotum and anus.

Peripheral zone: the part of the prostate gland in which prostate cancer usually starts to develop. It is also the part that usually becomes inflamed in prostatitis.

Phytotherapy: the use of plant extracts to combat illness, such as BPH.

PIN (prostatic intraepithelial neoplasia): the earliest stage in uncontrolled cell growth. It is not cancer, but is often a forerunner to it.

Prostatodynia: a state in which pain apparently comes from the prostate or surrounding area but there doesn't appear to be any inflammation or infection.

PSA (prostate-specific antigen): a substance made in the prostate gland that helps to liquefy the jelly-like storage form of sperm. If the prostate tissue becomes damaged or disrupted, as is particularly the case with prostate cancer, PSA leaks out into the bloodstream. As a consequence, blood levels of PSA tend to be higher among men with prostate cancer. A normal PSA value is taken as being below 4 ng/mL ('nanograms per millilitre').

Radical prostatectomy: an operation for prostate cancer in which the prostate, seminal vesicles and a sample of some nearby lymph nodes are removed. It is an option in fit men and only when the urologist believes that the cancer is still confined to the prostate.

Radiotherapy: the use of radiation to kill cancer cells. With external-beam radiotherapy, the radiation is generated from an external source and focused onto the area of the prostate. *See also* brachytherapy.

Recurrence: when the cancer begins to grow again after a period of dormancy.

Retrograde ejaculation: this occurs following some types of surgery on the prostate. Instead of semen passing out through the penis during orgasm, it passes into the bladder, from which it passes out of the body when the man urinates.

Risk factor: a personal characteristic that increases the likelihood of getting a certain disease. The effect of a **modifiable risk factor**, such as a high-fat diet or smoking, can be reduced or overcome, in contrast to a **non-modifiable risk factor** such as belonging to an older age group or having a first-degree relative with the disease.

Scrotum: the sac containing the testicles.

Seminal vesicles: storage vessels for sperm. They lie just behind the prostate and may be affected by prostate cancer as it spreads.

Staging system: a method used to assess and describe how far the cancer has spread. The **tumour–nodes–metastases (TNM) system** is commonly used in the UK.

Testicles (or testes): glands that make sperm and testosterone.

Testosterone: the hormone responsible for the development of many male characteristics. It has a role in stimulating growth of prostate tissue, so some of the drugs for prostate cancer and BPH work by disrupting its production or effect.

Tissue: a collection of cells organized into a structure that performs a specific function.

Transition zone: the part of the prostate in which BPH usually develops.

TRUS (transrectal ultrasonography): an ultrasound method that allows the prostate to be seen. It involves inserting a lubricated ultrasound probe into the rectum, and is often used during brachytherapy and biopsy procedures so that the radiotherapist or doctor can see the exact position of the patient's prostate.

TUIP (transurethral incision of the prostate): an operation for BPH in which small nicks are made in the neck of the bladder and in the prostate to relieve the pressure on the urethra.

TURP (transurethral resection of the prostate): an operation for BPH in which the middle of the enlarged prostate is cut away piecemeal using an instrument inserted up through the penis.

Ultrasound: a method of forming images using high-frequency sound waves.

Urethra: the tube that runs from the bladder to the tip of the penis, through which urine passes out from the body.

Urodynamics: a test to check how the bladder is functioning and whether the urine flow is blocked. It involves passing a fluid that will show up on X-rays into the bladder (via a catheter) and then recording the movement of this fluid while the patient urinates.

Uroflowmetry (urine flow test): a test to measure the speed of urine output over time. It involves the patient passing urine into a specialized receptacle called a **flow meter**.

Urologist: a doctor who has specialized in disorders affecting the kidney, bladder and, in men, the prostate.

Vas deferens: a tube that carries sperm from the testis to the prostate gland.

Vasopressin analogues: drugs that may be prescribed to reduce the need to pass urine at night.

How you can help Prostate Research Campaign UK

Research costs money, and large sums are needed to push forward the frontiers of knowledge and conquer diseases of the prostate. **Prostate Research Campaign UK** aims to provide information, promote education and raise funds to finance scientific and medical research into prostate disorders. Please do not leave the raising of funds to somebody else – everyone can help in some way. The need is undeniable.

Practical approaches

- You, or perhaps a group of friends, could help to raise money in your community through coffee mornings, sponsored walks, fun runs or some other type of popular event.

- Since April 2000, donations to charities have become tax efficient. Because **Prostate Research Campaign UK** is a registered charity it can recover tax on all donations that taxpayers make, providing that such donors sign a Gift Aid Declaration – forms are available from the address on page 107. Assuming a basic income tax rate of 22%, then for every £1 donated the charity can claim an additional 28 pence from the Inland Revenue. **Thus, for every £100 donated Prostate Research Campaign UK will receive an extra £28 at no extra cost to the donor**.

- If you are a higher rate taxpayer, you can also claim higher rate relief on payments made to charities under Gift Aid by including them on your self-assessment form. This relief is calculated at the difference between the basic rate and the higher rate of income tax on the gross value of the gift. For example, from £57 donated monthly, tax relief of £13 is available, making the actual cost to a donor paying a higher rate of tax £44. The value to the charity over 4 years on this example would be £3500.

- For companies wishing to make a donation, the procedure has been made simpler since April 2000. Companies can claim corporation tax relief on all donations to charities. For a company paying corporation tax at 30%, the **actual cost** of a gift of £1000 to **Prostate Research Campaign UK** would be only £700.

- From April 2000, gifts of publicly quoted shares, in addition to being exempt from capital gains tax liability, will enable the donor to claim income tax relief on the current value of the shares, which makes such gifts extremely tax efficient. For example, a higher rate taxpayer with a liability to pay capital gains tax, donating shares bought for £5000 and now worth £10,000, would save £2000 in capital gains tax and £4000 in income tax relief. So a gift worth £10,000 to **Prostate Research Campaign UK** would cost the donor just £4000.

- Please consider including a bequest to **Prostate Research Campaign UK** in your will. Your solicitor will advise on legacies made to charities when composing your will or a codicil to it. Please ensure that you check very carefully our charity registration number, which is 1037063, in the text.

- You will know that there are countless other ways of giving a charity the support it needs. Do please back the Campaign yourself and encourage others to support it too. Please send donations to the address below.

- Update is a regular newsletter distributed free by **Prostate Research Campaign UK**. It gives the latest information on research and treatments for all prostate conditions. Contact the address below to receive your copy.

Prostate Research Campaign UK
PO Box 2371, Swindon SN1 3WJ
Email: info@prostate-research.org.uk

Index